Plastic Surgery After Weight Loss

Editor

JEFFREY A. GUSENOFF

CLINICS IN PLASTIC SURGERY

www.plasticsurgery.theclinics.com

January 2019 • Volume 46 • Number 1

ELSEVIER

1600 John F. Kennedy Boulevard ● Suite 1800 ● Philadelphia, Pennsylvania, 19103-2899

http://www.theclinics.com

CLINICS IN PLASTIC SURGERY Volume 46, Number 1
January 2019 ISSN 0094-1298, ISBN-13: 978-0-323-65492-0

Editor: Jessica McCool
Developmental Editor: Meredith Madeira

Clinics in Plastic Surgery (ISSN 0094-1298) is published quarterly by Elsevier Inc., 360 Park Avenue South, New York, NY 10010-1710. Months of issue are January, April, July, and October. Business and Editorial Offices: 1600 John F. Kennedy Blvd., Suite 1800, Philadelphia, PA 19103-2899. Periodicals postage paid at New York, NY and additional mailing offices. Subscription prices are $543.00 per year for US individuals, $940.00 per year for US institutions, $100.00 per year for US students and residents, $607.00 per year for Canadian individuals, $1119.00 per year for Canadian institutions, $649.00 per year for international individuals, $1119.00 per year for international institutions, and $305.00 per year for Canadian and international students/residents. To receive student/resident rate, orders must be accompanied by name of affiliated institution, date of term, and the *signature* of program/residency coordinator on institution letterhead. Orders will be billed at individual rate until proof of status is received. Foreign air speed delivery is included in all *Clinics* subscription prices. All prices are subject to change without notice. **POSTMASTER:** Send address changes to *Clinics in Plastic Surgery*, Elsevier Health Sciences Division, Subscription Customer Service, 3251 Riverport Lane, Maryland Heights, MO 63043. **Customer Service: 1-800-654-2452 (US and Canada). From outside of the United States and Canada, call 314-447-8871. Fax: 314-447-8029. E-mail: JournalsCustomerService-usa@elsevier.com (for print support); JournalsOnlineSupport-usa@ elsevier.com (for online support).**

Reprints. For copies of 100 or more of articles in this publication, please contact the Commercial Reprints Department, Elsevier Inc., 360 Park Avenue South, New York, New York 10010-1710. Tel.: +1-212-633-3874; Fax: +1-212-633-3820; E-mail: reprints@elsevier.com.

Clinics in Plastic Surgery is covered in *Current Contents, EMBASE/Excerpta Medica, Science Citation Index, MEDLINE/ PubMed (Index Medicus), ASCA,* and *ISI/BIOMED.*

Contributors

EDITOR

JEFFREY A. GUSENOFF, MD
Professor, Department of Plastic Surgery,
University of Pittsburgh, Co-Director, UPMC
Life After Weight Loss Program, Pittsburgh,
Pennsylvania, USA

AUTHORS

TURKIA ABBED, MD
Hunstad Kortesis Bhartic Cosmetic Surgery,
Huntersville, North Carolina, USA

OMAR E. BEIDAS, MD
Body Contouring Fellow, Department of Plastic
and Reconstructive Surgery, University of
Pittsburgh Medical Center, Department of
Plastic Surgery, University of Pittsburgh,
Pittsburgh, Pennsylvania, USA

RONALD P. BOSSERT, MD
Director, Life After Weight Loss Program,
Associate Professor of Plastic Surgery,
Division of Plastic and Reconstructive Surgery,
University of Rochester Medical Center,
Rochester, New York, USA

JENNIFER CAPLA, MD
Private Practice, Department of Plastic
Surgery, Lenox Hill Hospital, Northwell Health
System, New York, New York, USA

CHARLIE CHEN, MD
Hunstad Kortesis Bharti Cosmetic Surgery,
Huntersville, North Carolina, USA

DEVIN COON, MD, MSE
Assistant Professor, Department of Plastic and
Reconstructive Surgery, Johns Hopkins
University, Baltimore, Maryland, USA

RAFAEL A. COUTO, MD
Department of Plastic Surgery, Dermatology
and Plastic Surgery Institute, Cleveland Clinic,
Cleveland, Ohio, USA

ALFREDO DONNABELLA, MD
Plastic Surgery Division, Botucatu Medical
School, Paulista State University, São Paulo,
Brazil

ALAN ROBERTO FAGOTTI MOREIRA, MD
Plastic Surgery Division, Botucatu Medical
School, Paulista State University, São Paulo,
Brazil

TALI FRIEDMAN, MD, MHA
The Body Contouring Center, Tel-Aviv, Israel

JEFFREY A. GUSENOFF, MD
Professor, Department of Plastic Surgery,
University of Pittsburgh, Co-Director, UPMC
Life After Weight Loss Program, Pittsburgh,
Pennsylvania, USA

MAARTEN HOOGBERGEN, MD, PhD
Department of Plastic and Reconstructive
Surgery, Catharina Hospital, Eindhoven, The
Netherlands

JOSEPH HUNSTAD, MD
President, Hunstad Kortesis Bharti Cosmetic
Surgery, Director, The American Society for
Aesthetic Plastic Surgery, Associate Clinical
Professor, Division of Plastic Surgery,
University of North Carolina at Chapel Hill,
Section Head, Plastic Surgery Carolinas
Medical Center, University Hospital, Charlotte,
North Carolina, USA

ANNE KLASSEN, DPhil
Department of Pediatrics, McMaster
University, Hamilton, Ontario, Canada

GEORGE KOKOSIS, MD
Resident, Department of Plastic and
Reconstructive Surgery, Johns Hopkins
University, Baltimore, Maryland, USA

GIANCARLO McEVENUE, MD
The McLean Clinic, Mississauga, Canada

FLÁVIO HENRIQUE MENDES, MD, PhD
Plastic Surgery Division, Botucatu Medical
School, Paulista State University, São Paulo,
Brazil

JOSEPH MICHAELS, MD
Private Practice, Michaels Aesthetic &
Reconstructive Plastic Surgery, North
Bethesda, Maryland, USA; Assistant Professor
of Plastic and Reconstructive Surgery, Johns
Hopkins Medicine, Baltimore, Maryland, USA

PAIGE L. MYERS, MD
Division of Plastic and Reconstructive Surgery,
University of Rochester Medical Center,
Rochester, New York, USA

DEEPAK NARAYAN, FRCS (Eng, Edin)
Section of Plastic and Reconstructive Surgery,
Department of Surgery, Yale School of
Medicine, New Haven, Connecticut, USA

AMANDA NORWICH, MD
Section of Plastic and Reconstructive Surgery,
Department of Surgery, Yale School of
Medicine, New Haven, Connecticut, USA

JEAN-FRANCOIS PASCAL, MD
Head of Scientific Council, IPSAC, Lyon,
France

LOTTE POULSEN, MD
Department of Plastic Surgery, Odense
University Hospital, Odense, Denmark

ANDREA PUSIC, MD, PhD
Department of Plastic and Reconstructive
Surgery, Brigham and Women's Hospital,
Harvard University, Boston, Massachusetts,
USA

J. PETER RUBIN, MD, FACS
Chair, Department of Plastic and
Reconstructive Surgery, University of
Pittsburgh Medical Center, Pittsburgh,
Pennsylvania, USA

LAUREN SHIKOWITZ-BEHR, MD
Department of Plastic Surgery, Lenox Hill
Hospital, Northwell Health System, Roslyn,
New York, USA

SANJA SLJIVIC, DO
Burn Surgery Fellow, Department of Surgery,
University of North Carolina, Chapel Hill,
North Carolina, USA

JENS AHM SORENSEN, MD, PhD
Department of Plastic Surgery, Odense
University Hospital, Odense, Denmark

JOSHUA T. WALTZMAN, MD, MBA
Private Practice, Waltzman Plastic and
Reconstructive Surgery, Long Beach,
California, USA

ITAY WISER, MD, PhD
Department of Epidemiology and Preventive
Medicine, Sackler Faculty of Medicine,
Tel-Aviv University, Tel-Aviv, Israel;
Department of Plastic Surgery, Lenox Hill
Hospital, New York, New York, USA

JAMES E. ZINS, MD
Chairman, Department of Plastic Surgery,
Dermatology and Plastic Surgery Institute,
Cleveland Clinic, Cleveland, Ohio, USA

Contents

The United States has experienced a significant increase in obesity over the past several decades, including a substantial increase in obesity-related comorbidities, such as type 2 diabetes, hypertension, heart disease, and obstructive sleep apnea. With obesity reaching epidemic proportions, there has been an increasing need for surgical intervention as a treatment option. Bariatric procedures have not only contributed to the significant weight loss a patient may experience but they have also had a profound effect on the decrease of weight-related comorbidities.

Comprehensive evaluation of the massive-weight-loss patient is a key factor to minimize complications while optimizing surgical outcomes. Special attention is given to medical and weight loss history, nutritional status, and physical examination. Massive-weight-loss patients often present with multiple areas of concern and therefore benefit from staged procedures. Staging requires knowledge on how the tissues are affected by each procedure and an understanding of the patient's priorities and goals.

Patient-reported outcome measures (PROMs) are questionnaires designed to measure outcomes of importance to patients from their perspective. The BODY-Q is a PROM designed to measure outcomes in weight loss and/or body contouring surgery. To develop the BODY-Q, a literature review, 63 patient interviews, 22 cognitive interviews, and input from 9 clinical experts were used to develop a conceptual framework that covers 3 broad domains: appearance concerns, health-related quality of life, and experience of care. For each aspect of the framework, multiple independently functioning scales were developed.

Body contouring after weight loss is becoming more prevalent. An appropriate systematic approach that starts from the first consultation needs to focus on residual comorbidities and weight of the patient. A thorough discussion about potential outcomes manages expectations. Preoperative optimization with smoking, herbal cessation, and nutritional assessment is mandatory. Planned staged approach minimizes lengthy procedures associated with increased postoperative morbidity. In the operating room, appropriate ambient temperature, positioning of the patient, and continuous discussion between surgeon and anesthesiologist prevent further complications. Careful transition to postoperative care with early ambulation and use of compressive garments add to an approach to minimize postoperative complications.

operation is tailored to the individual deformity, powerfully reshapes the breast, and can be safely combined with other commonly performed procedures. It is long-lasting and associated with minor complications that are easily treated in an office setting.

Bra-Line Back Lift

Joseph Hunstad, Charlie Chen, and Turkia Abbed

Upper back deformity caused by aging or fluctuations in weight are cosmetically and functionally unappealing to patients. Natural upper torso adherence zones create tether points that lead to horizontal and vertical laxity. Bra-line back lift is a versatile technique that can be used in any individual showing signs of redundant skin and adiposity. A 3-layered space-obliterating suture closure method prevents seroma and eliminates need for drain. Predictable outcomes correcting laxity from neck to lower back can be achieved. Gentle learning curve yields consistent and predictable results. Patient acceptance of the procedure, its results, and satisfactory morbidity rates have been universal.

Arm Contouring in the Massive-Weight-Loss Patient

Paige L. Myers and Ronald P. Bossert

Brachioplasty is an increasingly popular procedure performed for improved arm contour in the massive-weight-loss population. There are challenging deformities presented in this population, such as redundant skin, posterior arm lipodystrophy, and loosening of fascial layers of the upper arm and chest wall that must be addressed to achieve successful contour of the arms. Common complications can be minimized with meticulous technique and knowledge of surgical anatomy. Additionally, brachioplasty can be combined with liposuction of the posterior arm as a safe and effective method for arm contouring without a higher risk of complications.

Vertical Medial Thigh Contouring

Joseph Michaels

Excess thigh laxity is a problem for many patients following significant weight loss. Thigh laxity has both vertical and horizontal components that require correction to optimize the aesthetic appearance of the thigh. The vertical vector is best corrected first with a lower body lift or extended abdominoplasty. The remaining loose skin in the medial thigh can then be removed using a horizontal vector resulting in a vertical incision. Residual vertical skin excess is also removed parallel to the groin crease. This article describes the author's surgical approach and management of medial thigh deformity in the significant weight loss patient.

Face and Neck Lifting After Weight Loss

Joshua T. Waltzman, James E. Zins, and Rafael A. Couto

After massive weight loss, deflation of the tissues and loss of skin elasticity in the face and neck can result in the appearance of accelerated facial aging. Surgical facial rejuvenation can be successfully performed with several modifications. Proper preoperative counseling and expectation management regarding staged or ancillary procedures is recommended. Wide undermining of the face and neck, and extended postauricular incisions are required to allow for mobilization of excess skin and access to the mobile superficial musculoaponeurotic system (SMAS). Fat transfer into the deep malar compartment for midface volumizing is helpful. Treatment of the SMAS and platysma are universally necessary.

This article discusses strategies to prevent and manage the most common complications seen in body contouring surgery. General approaches to avoidance and treatment of these complications are addressed, including wound dehiscence, delayed wound healing, seroma, hematoma, infections of the surgical or remote sites, lymphedema, suture extrusion, and fat necrosis. Procedure-specific complications and pearls to avoiding complications in these cases are presented. Difficult problems, such as management of the disappointed patient, also are discussed.

CLINICS IN PLASTIC SURGERY

THE CLINICS ARE AVAILABLE ONLINE!
Access your subscription at:
www.theclinics.com

Preface
Body Contouring After Massive Weight Loss

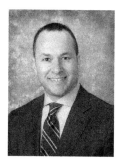

Jeffrey A. Gusenoff, MD
Editor

Body contouring after weight loss has become a growing niche in plastic surgery. Over the past decade, the rise in worldwide obesity has led to evolving trends in bariatric surgery that have a direct impact on the practice of plastic surgery. From banding procedures, to stomach plication, balloons, and sleeve procedures, there is a constant array of surgical and nonsurgical treatments aimed to combat the obesity epidemic. A major pitfall of massive weight loss is the significant skin relaxation that occurs afterwards. The excess skin makes patients feel uncomfortable, unhygienic, and in need for further improvement. Some even feel worse with the loose skin than when they were heavy. Patients then turn to plastic surgery to help complete the process of their weight loss journey with innovative procedures done in the safest manner.

The different procedures offered for body contouring after weight loss are numerous and include challenging operations like lower body lifts, back lifts, and thigh lifts that pose significant challenges. Additional areas that require new techniques or advances include the breasts, arms, face, and neck.

This issue of *Clinics in Plastic Surgery* covers many key areas of the subspecialty, including a review of the scope of management of the obesity epidemic, patient evaluation prior to body contouring with an emphasis on patient safety, how to stage patients appropriately, and how to perform state-of-the-art techniques by world leaders in the field. This issue also covers important topics of pain control in body contouring procedures as well as a comprehensive understanding of complications that can arise and how to manage or avoid them.

I am very appreciative of the work of all the contributors for this issue; without their efforts and dedication, this collection would not be possible. It is wonderful to have such excellent minds and technically gifted surgeons in the field of body contouring, constantly working to evolve the field and improve outcomes for this special population. I hope this international collection of authors provides a well-rounded review of the field of body contouring today, provides insight into the challenges of body contouring, and opens the door to future innovations in the field.

Jeffrey A. Gusenoff, MD
University of Pittsburgh
3380 Boulevard of the Allies, Suite 180
Pittsburgh, PA 15213, USA

E-mail address:
gusenoffja@upmc.edu

Clin Plastic Surg 46 (2019) xi
https://doi.org/10.1016/j.cps.2018.09.001
0094-1298/19/© 2018 Published by Elsevier Inc.

The Obesity Epidemic and Bariatric Trends

Sanja Sljivic, DO[a], Jeffrey A. Gusenoff, MD[b],*

KEYWORDS

- Obesity • United States • Epidemic • Population health • Bariatric surgery
- Laparoscopic sleeve gastrectomy • Gastric bypass

KEY POINTS

- Prevalence of obesity (body mass index >30 kg/m^2) has increased drastically in the United States since the 1990s.
- In 2013, the American Medical Association recognized obesity as a disease.
- The annual medical costs of obesity were estimated to be $40 billion in 2006.
- The most common bariatric procedures in the United States are gastric banding, sleeve gastrectomy, and gastric bypass.
- Patients undergoing bariatric surgery may lose significant amounts of excess weight and experience improvement in obesity-related comorbidities.

INTRODUCTION

Despite efforts at prevention, the prevalence of obesity in the United States has reached 30% in most adult age groups.[1] In 2013, the American Medical Association officially recognized obesity as a disease, stirring up a debate within the medical community. Those who supported this decision argued that the new classification would place more emphasis on this health problem among physicians and insurance companies, whereas others claimed that the stigma of being diagnosed with a disease would be even greater. However, it became clear that obesity was no longer simply a developing health issue within the medical community, but rather, it had reached epidemic levels both in the United States and globally.[2]

THE OBESITY EPIDEMIC IN NUMBERS
Defining Obesity

Body mass index (BMI) is the most common and most widely used tool to quantify obesity, and it is calculated using the following formula[3]:

$$\frac{weight\ (lb)}{[height\ (in)]^2} \times 703$$

It has been shown that BMI is a strong predictor of overall mortality and is directly associated with the presence of comorbidities.[4] An individual is considered obese if their BMI is greater than 30 kg/m^2, with this further classified into 3 grades of obesity (**Table 1**).[3]

Trends in Obesity

The US Department of Health and Human Services launched "Healthy People 2010" in January 2000, which was a nationwide disease prevention campaign. In collaboration with the Food and Drug Administration and the National Institutes of Health (NIH), the objective was to promote health and reduce chronic disease associated with obesity in the United States.[4] The following objectives were to be achieved by 2010:

1. Increase the number of US adults who are at a healthy weight (BMI between 18.5 and 25 kg/m^2) from 42% to 60%

Disclosure Statement: The authors have nothing to disclose.
[a] Department of Surgery, University of North Carolina, 4001 Burnett-Womack Building, CB #7050, Chapel Hill, NC 27599-7050, USA; [b] Department of Plastic Surgery, University of Pittsburgh, 3380 Boulevard of the Allies, Suite 180, Pittsburgh, PA 15213, USA
* Corresponding author.
E-mail address: gusenoffja@upmc.edu

Clin Plastic Surg 46 (2019) 1–7
https://doi.org/10.1016/j.cps.2018.08.001

Table 1 Weight range classification	
	BMI (kg/m²)
Underweight	<18.5
Normal weight range	18.5–24.9
Overweight	25–29.9
Obesity	>30
Grade I	30–34.9
Grade II	35–39.9
Grade III (morbid obesity)	>40

Data from National Heart, Lung and Blood Institute, National Institute of Diabetes and Digestive and Kidney Diseases (U.S.). Clinical guidelines on the identification, evaluation, and treatment of overweight and obesity in adults: the evidence report. Bethesda (MD): National Institutes of Health, National Heart, Lung and Blood Institute; 1998.

2. Decrease the number of US adults who are obese (BMI >30 kg/m²) from 23% to 15%
3. Decrease the number of US children and adolescents who are overweight or obese from 11% to 5%[4]

However, data obtained from the same source between 2007 and 2008 demonstrated that none of these objectives had been met. In fact, the following numbers were noted:

1. The number of US adults who were considered to be at a healthy weight decreased from 42% to 32%
2. The number of US adults who were considered obese increased from 23% to 33.8%
3. The number of overweight or obese children and adolescents in the US increased from 11% to 16.9%[4]

These numbers not only showed the magnitude of obesity as a disease but also presented a daunting task to those working to reverse the current trend.

The Centers for Disease Control and Prevention (CDC) studied this issue further via the National Health and Nutrition Examination Survey and found that the prevalence of obesity was higher among women than men overall (**Fig. 1**), and higher among African American and Hispanic adults (**Fig. 2**).[5]

In addition, the CDC collected state data about US residents' health-related risk behaviors and chronic health conditions via the Behavioral Risk Factor Surveillance System (BRFSS). Each year, about 400,000 telephone interviews are completed, making this a powerful tool for both obtaining behavioral health risk data in terms of

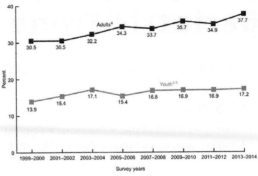

Fig. 1. Trends in obesity prevalence among adults aged 20 and over and youth aged 2 to 19 years in the United States, 1999 to 2000 through 2013 to 2014. All estimates are age adjusted to the 2000 US census population using age groups 20 to 39, 40 to 59, and 60 and over. ([a] Significant increasing linear trend from 1999–2000 through 2013–2014. [b] Test for linear trend for 2003–2004 through 2013–2014 not significant [*P*>.05]. All adult estimates are age adjusted by the direct method to the 2000 US census population using the age groups 20 to 39, 40 to 59, and 60 and over.) (*From* Ogden CL, Carroll MD, Fryar CD, et al. Prevalence of obesity among adults and youth: United States, 2011–2014. NCHS Data Brief, No. 219. Hyattsville (MD): National Center for Health Statistics; 2015; with permission.)

obesity and creating health promotion activities. One of the most significant forms of data obtained is the prevalence of self-reported obesity among US adults (**Fig. 3**).[6]

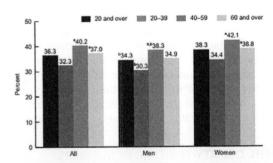

Fig. 2. Prevalence of obesity among adults aged 20 and over distributed by sex, race, and Hispanic origin in the United States, 2011 to 2014. All estimates are age adjusted to the 2000 US census population using age groups 20 to 39, 40 to 59, and 60 and over. ([a] Significantly different from those aged 20–39. [b] Significantly different from women of the same age group. Totals were age adjusted by the direct method to the 2000 US census population using the age groups 20–39, 40–59, and 60 and over. Crude estimates are 36.5% for all, 34.5% for men, and 38.5% for women.) (*From* Ogden CL, Carroll MD, Fryar CD, et al. Prevalence of obesity among adults and youth: United States, 2011–2014. NCHS Data Brief, No. 219. Hyattsville (MD): National Center for Health Statistics; 2015; with permission.)

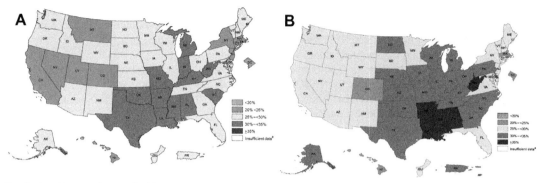

Fig. 3. BRFSS: prevalence of self-reported obesity among US adults by state and territory in (*A*) 2011 and (*B*) 2016. Obesity is defined as BMI $\geq$30.0 kg/m^2; BMI was calculated from self-reported weight and height. Respondents that were excluded included those with weight less than 50 pounds or $\geq$650 pounds; height less than 3 feet or $\geq$8 feet; or BMI less than 12 or $\geq$100. Pregnant respondents were also excluded. [a]Sample size <50 or the relative standard error (dividing the standard error by the prevalence) $\geq$ 30%. (*From* CDC Behavioral Risk Factor Surveillance System. Prevalence of self-reported obesity among U.S. adults by state and territory. Available at: http://www.cdc.gov/obesity/data/prevalence-maps.html. Accessed January 3, 2018.)

The Cost of Obesity

The alarming rates of obesity in the United States have created a significant public health concern and a substantial financial burden on our society. Several studies have attempted to estimate the costs of obesity, with some reporting the annual medical costs to be $40 billion in 2006.[7] Other studies have used an instrumental variable approach, which uses genetic variation in weight as a natural experiment, to show that the estimated medical costs of obesity could reach $209.7 billion.[8] These results, however, may not be generalizable to the entire population because the study was restricted to adults aged 20 to 64 years with biological children aged 11 to 20 years.[1,8]

More recently, a systematic review was published in 2016, concentrating on the most current literature regarding costs of obesity. The investigators found that the pooled estimate of annual medical costs of obesity was $1901 in 2014, thus accounting for $149.4 billion at the national level. They also noted that one of the main limitations of estimating costs associated with obesity was the lack of distinction between cost of obesity related to comorbidities versus cost of obesity care itself.[1] Although there appears to be some variation among the estimates, it still remains clear that obesity is a costly public health concern.

GUIDELINES FOR QUALIFICATION FOR BARIATRIC SURGERY

According to the American Society for Metabolic and Bariatric Surgery (ASMBS), bariatric procedures should be provided as an option to 2 groups:

1. Patients with a BMI greater than 40 kg/m^2 or more without coexisting medical problems for whom surgery would not be associated with increased risk
2. Patients with a BMI greater than 35 kg/m^2 or more with one or more obesity-related comorbidities[9]

The use of bariatric surgery worldwide is largely governed by an NIH consensus statement published 22 years ago. Although these guidelines have been valuable, they are somewhat outdated and present significant limitations. For instance, only open procedures were considered, whereas most procedures nowadays are performed laparoscopically. Also, these guidelines provided only limited recommendations for diabetes; however, over the years, it has become obvious that bariatric procedures exert significant effects on type 2 diabetes.[10]

Even though surgical options have evolved greatly since the original NIH recommendations were written, surgical practice has been guided by them. They have provided us with extensive clinical evidence, thereby validating the use of these guidelines in making treatment decisions for severely obese patients. Studies examining thousands of participants for up to 20 years show that, among such individuals, bariatric surgery is associated with a long-term decrease in most obesity-related comorbidities, including cardiovascular disease, strokes, and cancer.[10]

TYPES OF BARIATRIC PROCEDURES

The best choice for any bariatric surgery depends on the goals of therapy for each individual patient (eg, weight loss and/or glycemic control), expertise of the surgeon and institution, patient preferences, and personalized risk stratification. In general, laparoscopic bariatric procedures are preferred over open procedures due to lower early postoperative morbidity and mortality.[9]

The most common weight-loss procedures in the United States (**Fig. 4**) include adjustable gastric banding (AGB), sleeve gastrectomy (SG), and Roux-en-Y gastric bypass (RYGB). Another procedure that is less commonly performed includes biliopancreatic diversion with duodenal switch (BPD-DS). This particular surgery has fallen out of favor over the years secondary to high complication rates.[11] The ASMBS has estimated that more than 200,000 bariatric procedures are performed each year, with SG procedures exceeding the number of RYGB procedures (**Table 2**).[11,12]

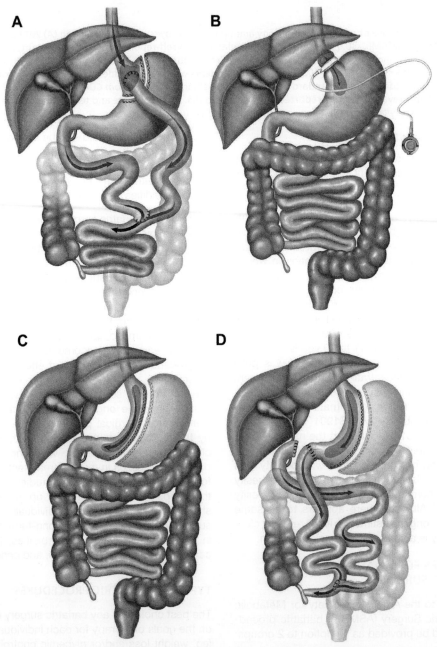

Fig. 4. Types of bariatric procedures: (*A*) RYGB ; (*B*) AGB; (*C*) SG; (*D*) BPD-DS. (*Courtesy of* © Ethicon, Inc. 2018. Reproduced with permission.)

Table 2
Percentage breakdown of bariatric procedures in the United States, 2011 to 2016

	2011	2012	2013	2014	2015	2016
Total	158,000	173,000	179,000	193,000	196,000	216,000
AGB (%)	35.4	20.2	14	9.5	5.7	3.4
SG (%)	17.8	33	42.1	51.7	53.8	58.1
RYGB (%)	36.7	37.5	34.2	26.8	23.1	18.7
BPD-DS (%)	0.9	1	1	0.4	0.6	0.6

Data from English WJ, DeMaria EJ, Brethauer SA, et al. American Society for Metabolic and Bariatric Surgery estimation of metabolic and bariatric procedures performed in the United States in 2016. Surg Obes Relat Dis 2017. https://doi.org/10.1016/j.soard.2017.12.013.

Adjustable Gastric Banding

AGB procedures are mainly characterized by reversibility and low incidence of procedure-related complications; however, the number of these procedures performed each year has decreased in recent years. The decrease in bands appears to be mainly due to variability in weight loss and lower effectiveness in decreasing weight-related comorbidities.[11]

In AGB, a band that contains an inflatable silastic balloon is placed around the proximal stomach. This band, which is located below the gastroesophageal junction, can be tightened via a subcutaneous access port by injecting or withdrawing a saline solution.[13]

Roux-en-Y Gastric Bypass

RYGB has been performed since its development in the 1960s. It has withstood the test of time because of its durability and effectiveness in achieving long-term weight loss and comorbidity reduction. The procedure was performed initially using an open surgical technique, which ultimately contributed to a higher incidence of wound-related complications. Today, it can be performed safely by experienced surgeons using a laparoscopic approach.[11]

In RYGB, the stomach is divided into an upper gastric pouch and a lower gastric remnant. The gastric pouch holds about 15 to 30 mL in volume and is anastomosed to the jejunum after it has been divided about 30 to 75 cm distal to the ligament of Treitz. This distal portion is brought up as a "Roux limb," whereas the excluded biliary limb is connected to the bowel about 75 to 150 cm distal to the gastrojejunostomy.[13]

Sleeve Gastrectomy

SG was initially performed as a first-stage procedure in BPD-DS; however, over the years, SG has gained popularity as a stand-alone operation secondary to the high complication rates of BPD-DS.[11]

In SG, the stomach is transected vertically over a bougie, thereby creating a gastric tube and leaving a 100- to 200-mL pouch.[13] The portion of the stomach that is resected results in both reduced gastric capacity and Ghrelin output, thereby controlling a patient's hunger.[11]

Several studies have examined the effects of bougie size on both complication rates (eg, strictures, leaks) and ultimate weight loss results. A survey performed in 2014 found that the most common bougie size was 36 French, which was used by 38.4% of the surgeons surveyed.[14]

Biliopancreatic Diversion with Duodenal Switch

BPD-DS is mainly a malabsorptive operation with favorable surgical results; however, this comes at the expense of higher postoperative complications, including malnutrition and vitamin/mineral deficiencies.[11]

In BPD-DS, a vertical SG is created and the transection of the duodenum is performed just beyond the pylorus. The alimentary limb is then connected to the duodenum, whereas the biliopancreatic limb is anastomosed to the ileum about 75 cm proximal to the ileocecal valve.[13]

TRENDS IN BARIATRIC SURGERY

Between 2008 and 2012, more than 500,000 bariatric procedures were performed within the United States. Khan and colleagues[9] observed an overall decrease in the number of bariatric operations performed during that 4-year period; however, there was an observed increase of procedures from 2011 to 2012. The number of laparoscopic sleeve gastrectomies increased more than 5 times from 8.2% of all bariatric procedures in 2011 to 39.6% in 2012. The use of AGB decreased from 28.8% in 2008 to 5.6% in 2012. Open gastric bypass procedures were the least commonly performed procedures overall.

Sleeve Gastrectomy Versus Roux-en-Y Gastric Bypass

SG procedures are generally considered to be technically easier, faster to perform, and potentially safer than RYGB procedures; however, there appears to be more data on clinical and metabolic long-term outcomes of RYGB than SG. Until this point, the limited number of randomized studies that have been performed mainly included low patient numbers and short follow-up.[15]

Recently, however, 2 randomized clinical trials were published after evaluating the effects of laparoscopic SG versus laparoscopic RYGB on weight loss in patients with morbid obesity.[15,16] The Swiss Multicenter Bypass or Sleeve Study (SM-BOSS) and the Sleeve versus Bypass (SLEEVE-PASS) trial both involved morbidly obese patients, who were randomized to undergo either laparoscopic SG or laparoscopic RYGB. The primary endpoint of these studies was weight loss evaluated by percentage excess BMI loss,[16] whereas secondary endpoints included resolution of comorbidities.[15,16]

After 5 years, the SM-BOSS study did not find any significant difference in percentage of excess BMI loss when comparing patients who underwent either laparoscopic SG or RYGB. In addition, obesity-related comorbidities (eg, type 2 diabetes and dyslipidemia) were reduced after both procedures, with the exception of gastroesophageal reflux disease (GERD), which was achieved more often after RYGB. In fact, worsening of GERD was more common among patients who underwent SG. In terms of dyslipidemia, the study found no significant difference in total cholesterol, high-density lipoprotein cholesterol (HDL-C), or triglycerides between the groups; however, the ratio of total cholesterol to HDL-C and low-density lipoprotein cholesterol (LDL-C) was significantly better 5 years after RYGB.[16]

In the SLEEVEPASS study, both laparoscopic SG and RYGB procedures resulted in sustained weight loss, with a mean excess weight loss of 49% in the SG group and 57% in the RYGB group. However, even though RYGB was associated with greater percentage weight loss at 5 years, the confidence interval extended both above and below the equivalence margin, and thus, no conclusions could be made about whether RYGB was superior to SG from a clinical standpoint. There was no statistically significant difference between SG and RYGB for type 2 diabetes remission or dyslipidemia resolution. However, LDL-C levels were found to be lower in patients who underwent RYGB than those in the SG group. In terms of lack of type 2 diabetes resolution, the investigators attributed this to possible differences in preoperative diabetes duration, because shorter diabetes duration at baseline would be associated with more favorable remission rates after bariatric surgery.[15]

LOOKING AHEAD

Bariatric surgery not only induces weight loss but also improves weight-related comorbidities such as diabetes and dyslipidemia.[15,16] Recent changes in surgical trends demonstrate that the field of bariatric surgery is actively changing. Presently, SG appears to be dominating the procedural milieu,[17] although studies such as the SM-BOSS and SLEEVEPASS trials have not demonstrated significant differences in weight loss between SG and RYGB.[15,16]

It is very likely that obesity and diabetes will be increasingly treated via surgical and even endoscopic procedures. Bariatric care will continue to be a growing field for surgeons and therapeutic endoscopists with many future opportunities for expansion, innovation, and improvement.[17]

REFERENCES

1. Kim DD, Basu A. Estimating the medical care costs of obesity in the United States: systematic review, meta-analysis, and empirical analysis. Value Health 2016;19(5):602–13.
2. Ortiz SE, Kawachi I, Boyce AM. The medicalization of obesity, bariatric surgery, and population health. Health (London) 2016;21(5):498–518.
3. National Heart, Lung and Blood Institute, National Institute of Diabetes and Digestive and Kidney Diseases (U.S.). Clinical guidelines on the identification, evaluation, and treatment of overweight and obesity in adults: the evidence report. Bethesda (MD): National Institutes of Health, National Heart, Lung and Blood Institute; 1998.
4. Azagury DE, Lautz DB. Obesity overview: epidemiology, health and financial impact, and guidelines for qualification for surgical therapy. Gastrointest Endosc Clin N Am 2011;21(2):189–201.
5. Ogden CL, Carroll MD, Fryar CD, et al. Prevalence of obesity among adults and youth: United States, 2011-2014. NCHS Data Brief, No. 219. Hyattsville (MD): National Center for Health Statistics; 2015.
6. CDC – Behavioral Risk Factor Surveillance System. Prevalence of self-reported obesity among U.S. adults by state and territory. Available at: http://www.cdc.gov/obesity/data/prevalence-maps.html. Accessed January 3, 2018.
7. Finkelstein EA, Trogdon JG, Cohen JW, et al. Annual medical spending attributable to obesity: payer- and service-specific estimates. Health Aff 2009;28(5):w822–31.

8. Cawley J, Meyerhoefer C. The medical care costs of obesity: an instrumental variables approach. J Health Econ 2012;31:219–30.

9. Khan S, Rock K, Baskara A, et al. Trends in bariatric surgery from 2008 to 2012. Am J Surg 2016;211(6): 1041–6.

10. Cummings DE, Cohen RV. Beyond BMI: the need for new guidelines governing the use of bariatric and metabolic surgery. Lancet Diabetes Endocrinol 2014;2(2):175–81.

11. Bour ES. Evidence supporting the need for bariatric surgery to address the obesity epidemic in the United States. Curr Sports Med Rep 2015;14(2):100–3.

12. English WJ, DeMaria EJ, Brethauer SA, et al. American Society for Metabolic and Bariatric Surgery estimation of metabolic and bariatric procedures performed in the United States in 2016. Surg Obes Relat Dis 2018;14(3):259–63.

13. Neff KJ, Olbers T, Le Roux CW. Bariatric surgery: the challenges with candidate selection, individualizing treatment and clinical outcomes. BMC Med 2013; 11(1):8.

14. Gagner M, Hutchinson C, Rosenthal R. Fifth international consensus conference: current status of sleeve gastrectomy. Surg Obes Relat Dis 2016; 12(4):750–6.

15. Salminen P, Helmiö M, Ovaska J, et al. Effect of laparoscopic sleeve gastrectomy vs laparoscopic Roux-en-Y gastric bypass on weight loss at 5 years among patients with morbid obesity: the SLEEVEPASS randomized clinical trial. JAMA 2018;319(3): 241–54.

16. Peterli R, Wölnerhanssen BK, Peters T, et al. Effect of laparoscopic sleeve gastrectomy vs laparoscopic Roux-en-Y gastric bypass on weight loss in patients with morbid obesity: the SM-BOSS randomized clinical trial. JAMA 2018;319(3):255–65.

17. Roslin MS, Cripps C, Peristeri A. Bariatric and metabolic surgery: current trends and what's to follow. Curr Opin Gastroenterol 2015;31(6):513–8.

Patient Evaluation and Surgical Staging

Jennifer Capla, MD[a],*, Lauren Shikowitz-Behr, MD[b]

KEYWORDS

• Massive weight loss • Post–bariatric • BMI • Body contouring • Staging

KEY POINTS

- In order to properly evaluate the massive-weight-loss patient, a complete medical workup focusing on medical comorbidities, weight history, and nutritional status must be performed.
- A comprehensive physical examination is key: evaluate body habitus, skin excess, and skin quality; Distinguish between intraperitoneal and subcutaneous fat; determine which areas are of greatest concern and consider debulking liposuction at the first stage to improve second-stage excision results; understand how vectors of pull can impact outcomes, and review which procedures are best combined and which should be avoided.
- Patients who desire correction of multiple areas will require staging. Consider the patient's goals and try to address their priorities as the first operation. Managing patient expectations is important. Tradeoff includes significant scarring for an improved contour.

INTRODUCTION

The key to successful body contouring after massive weight loss is proper patient selection and an understanding of how to combine and stage procedures. Patients often present with multiple areas of concern. All areas should be assessed, but understanding the patient's priorities and goals is a key factor to patient satisfaction. It is the plastic surgeon's responsibility to achieve optimal aesthetic outcomes while limiting complications. Staging procedures helps to minimize operative time, decrease complications, and ensure that procedures do not compromise aesthetic outcome with opposition of pull.

EVALUATION OF THE MASSIVE-WEIGHT-LOSS PATIENT

Comprehensive evaluation of the weight loss patient is a key component to minimizing complications. Characteristics of the post–bariatric surgery population deviate significantly from those of the non-weight loss body contouring patients. Evaluation should include standard medical and surgical history with special attention to the weight loss history, including:

Maximum weight and maximum body mass index (BMI) max
Current weight and BMI
Total weight loss
Length of stable weight
Goal weight
Type of weight loss surgery (restrictive or malabsorptive)

As a general guideline, BMI at or less than 30 kg/m^2 is accepted as a safe cutoff for selecting candidates to undergo post–bariatric body contouring procedures. High BMI (>30) is associated with increased postoperative complications. In addition, patients who have achieved a greater weight loss or a higher delta BMI are at risk for greater postsurgical issues.[1–4]

The authors have nothing to disclose.
a Department of Plastic Surgery, Lenox Hill Hospital, Northwell Health System, 125 East 63rd Street, New York, NY 10065, USA; b Department of Plastic Surgery, Lenox Hill Hospital, Northwell Health System, 48 Chestnut Hill, Roslyn, NY 11576, USA
* Corresponding author.
E-mail address: jennifer.capla@gmail.com

Clin Plastic Surg 46 (2019) 9–14
https://doi.org/10.1016/j.cps.2018.08.002

Weight stability is another essential component to the weight loss history. Patients must have a stable weight for at least 3 months, defined as no more than a 5-pound weight loss per month for 3 consecutive months, to consider body contouring. Many prefer 6 months; however, 3 months is the minimum.[5] During that time, many medical comorbidities resolve, and new physiologic homeostasis is achieved. In addition, if the weight is stable, the results of body contouring will be optimized.

MEDICAL COMORBIDITIES

Overweight and obese individuals have an increased incidence of heart disease, diabetes mellitus, sleep apnea, osteoarthritis, lipid abnormalities, and hypertension, among a multitude of other medical problems. Although weight loss alone may lessen or even cure some health issues, there is often lingering disease requiring assessment and management. Any medical conditions that are not resolved after weight loss must receive a proper workup. Inquire about changes in medication dosage and any changes in symptoms.

Skin redundancy contributes to additional comorbid conditions, including musculoskeletal pain, infections and rashes, difficulty with ambulation and sexual activity, and complex psychological issues, including depression.[6] Consider consulting with a psychiatrist for a mental health workup as part of the preoperative routine. Mental stability is critical for withstanding the physical and emotional stressors of massive weight loss and the recovery process from staged body contouring procedures.

NUTRITIONAL STATUS

Nutritional deficiencies are common in the bariatric surgery and massive-weight-loss populations. Procedures like the Roux-en-Y gastric bypass cause a malabsorptive physiology leading to micronutrient deficits. Iron deficiency is noted in up to 50% of the post–bariatric surgery population, sometimes leading to iron deficiency anemia. Deficiencies in calcium, vitamin B12, and thiamine are all linked to this patient population.[7] In addition, protein malnutrition can be multifactorial after bariatric surgery, and although this may be inconsequential in a nonstressed state, protein malnutrition post operatively it can lead to delayed recovery and poor wound healing. All weight loss patients should be assessed for nutritional status and optimized with a nutritionist before surgery.

SMOKING CESSATION

Smoking has been shown to increase postoperative complications, including delayed wound healing. Patients with a smoking history are required to abstain for at least 4 weeks before and 4 weeks after surgery. The surgeon should defer surgery on active smokers.

SOCIAL SUPPORT

Having a strong social support network is advantageous for patients undergoing body contouring surgery, especially when staged surgery is planned. Physical limitations during the recovery phase require assistance with activities of daily living. Special considerations should be given to patients undergoing brachioplasty who have difficulty using their arms, and patients who undergo thigh lifts and may have difficulty with ambulation. It is also important to encourage proper nutrition, hygiene, and adherence to medication regimens.

PHYSICAL EXAMINATION

Perform a thorough physical examination. Evaluate for body shape and habitus. Distinguish between prevalent subcutaneous or intraperitoneal fat. Assess for skin rolls and redundant tissues; pinch tissues to measure skin quality and elasticity and specifically if they have more skin laxity versus underlying fatty tissue. An overhanging pannus or ptotic breasts may hide intertriginous rashes and/or open wounds. While examining the abdomen, be sure to note prior surgical scars and the presence of hernias and palpate for rectus diastasis. The authors recommend assessing the patient's skin laxity versus their excess subcutaneous fat, and consider if liposuction during the first stage would benefit results of the second.

PATIENT EXPECTATIONS

Managing patient expectations is perhaps the most important part of the body contouring surgery journey. Weight loss patients often present for consultation with multiple areas of concern. A patient must understand that not all procedures can be performed at one time, and staging is necessary. With the patient standing in front of a mirror, use a skin displacement or a pinch technique to demonstrate the power of each procedure. Just as important, the limitations of the procedures must be pointed out as well. Patients will have to accept extensive scarring in exchange for contour. Location and quality of the scars should be discussed in detail because this is one of the larger tradeoffs for patients. When discussing the patient's options, careful attention to the patient's goals should be considered. A patient's top priorities should be targeted in the first procedure if deemed appropriate.

STAGING IN BODY CONTOURING SURGERY

Massive-weight-loss patients often desire correction of multiple areas. Body contouring procedures can therefore be lengthy and labor intensive. Staging is an important component to obtaining the best cosmetic results while decreasing postoperative complications. In order to minimize complications, there are several factors to consider.

Patient Safety

Patient safety should always be the top priority. Although there is no absolute rule for the length of duration for general anesthesia in elective surgery, a 6-hour limit is routinely accepted. A 6-hour limit is particularly true when body contouring is performed in the outpatient ambulatory surgery setting. As the volume of body contouring surgery increases, many surgeons are performing these operations in an outpatient setting. In this case, several factors contribute to safety and efficacy, including American Society of Anesthesiologists class 1 or 2, operative time less than 6 hours, and limiting lipoaspirate to 2 L when combined with other surgical procedures. It has been shown that duration of surgery is an independent predictor of complications, with a significantly increased risk as cases become longer than 3 hours.[8,9] In addition, one must keep in mind that, with each additional procedure performed, the risk of wound-healing complications increases.

Operative Team

When combining multiple surgeries in a single stage, consider the availability of an assistant surgeon to limit fatigue. If a 2-team approach is possible, this will decrease the overall operative time. Involve the perioperative team in planning and discussion, including the operating room nurse, surgical scrub, and anesthesiologist.[10] It is important to have a team that understands these cases. At times, prepping and draping the patient for multiple procedures is a challenge. Knowing where to allow the anesthesiologist to place their monitors and blood pressure cuff, instructing the location of the Bovie grounding pads, Sequential Compression Device boots, and appropriate padding for positioning and turns requires thought and preparation in advance.

Patient Priorities

When considering staging, it is important to keep a patient's priorities and goals in mind. Even with planned staging, always try to target the top priority in the first stage. It is important to listen to the patient and understand what they desire to achieve.

Combinations of Procedures

There are several options of body contouring procedures that can be combined into one operation. Which is the best combination will vary from surgeon to surgeon. However, there are some guidelines on how to select these combinations. These guidelines are reviewed as some of the more common combinations are discussed (**Figs. 1** and **2**).

Abdominoplasty/Breast Procedure

The abdominoplasty/breast procedure is the most common combination of body contouring procedures performed in the non-weight-loss population and therefore has translated over. A traditional abdominoplasty is performed along with any hernia repairs. The type of breast procedure will vary but may include a mastopexy, reduction, augmentation, or gynecomastia correction. The massive-weight-loss breast deformity is distinct and technically challenging to correct compared with the non-weight-loss population. Therefore, this is not a common combination in the authors' practice unless a patient desires it in a single stage.

Time: This procedure is performed entirely in the supine position, eliminating time lost on turns.

Caveat: "Fixed" structures like the inframammary fold (IMF) of the breast may be loose and easily displaced in the massive-weight-loss patient. In a traditional abdominoplasty, it may displace the IMF in a downward direction. If performing a fleur-de-lis (FDL) abdominoplasty, then there is the added concern of a medial pull on the IMF.

Abdominoplasty/Lower Body Lift ± Brachioplasty

The abdominoplasty/lower body lift (LBL) combination focuses on the midsection in a circumferential fashion. It targets the excess skin of the abdomen, mons ptosis, lateral thigh, and buttock ptosis. An abdominoplasty and LBL can be performed separately, but when combined, it helps to eliminate dog ears and allows for greater excision of the lateral abdominal tissues.

Time: This procedure must start prone. That means that there are 2 flips to consider when calculating operative time. In addition, if considering an abdominoplasty with a FDL and/or a gluteal autoaugmentation, this will add a significant amount of time to the procedure. If that is

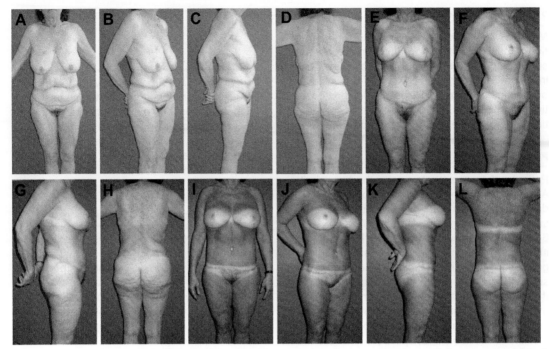

Fig. 1. A 58-year-old woman following 73 kg (160 lb) weight loss from roux-en-Y gastric bypass who desired dermal suspension mastopexy and abdominoplasty, a combination of procedures that is generally favorable, and brachioplasty. Preoperative photographs (*A–D*) and postoperative photographs at 1 year (*E–H*) are shown. No significant change in buttock or trunk contour is effected form this combination, as expected. The patient returned desiring additional body contouring of the buttock and trunk. A second stage circumferential body lift was performed and the scars merged with the abdominoplasty scars, along with a limited lateral chest transverse resection to correct upper trunk contour. If a full transverse upper body lift was planned, it would have been staged relative to the lower body lift to avoid opposing vectors of tension. Postoperative photos are shown 2 years after the first stage (*I–L*). (*From* Capla J, Rubin JP. Staging and combining procedures. In: Rubin JP, editor. Body contouring and liposuction. Saunders; 2013. p. 593–603, with permission.)

the case, consider eliminating the brachioplasty from this stage.

Caveat: Patient recovery. When plicating the rectus abdominis muscles, patients will have a difficult time using their rectus muscles to sit up, which means they are reliant on their arms to help pull them up. This fact is something to make patients aware of for the recovery period.

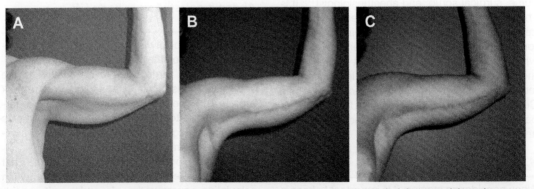

Fig. 2. Brachioplasty photographs for the patient in Fig. 55.1 shown preoperatively (*A*), 1 year (*B*), and two years (*C*) postoperatively demonstrating maturation of the bicipital groove scar. (*From* Capla J, Rubin JP. Staging and combining procedures. In: Rubin JP, editor. Body contouring and liposuction. Saunders; 2013. p. 593–603, with permission.)

Breast Procedure/Upper Body Lift ± Brachioplasty

The benefit of a circumferential procedure is to eliminate dog ears and to improve the aesthetic results by allowing additional excess skin excision. Therefore, it is always preferable to pair procedures that allow contouring 360°.

Time: This procedure must start prone. That means that there are 2 flips to consider when calculating operative time.

Caveat: If performing an autoaugmentation of the breast with the lateral midaxillary tissue rolls, be sure to mark this clearly in advance, because it can easily be excised during the upper body lift (UBL). If a UBL is done with another procedure before breast, be careful not to excise the lateral rolls because this option will be eliminated for future use.

Vertical Medial Thigh Lift

This procedure targets the loose skin of the medial thighs. It can be combined with any of the upper body procedures. Generally, for the best aesthetic outcome, it should not be combined with but rather should proceed an abdominoplasty/LBL. The effect of these procedures on the medial thighs would be an upward and lateral pull, respectively, working in opposition to the medial pull of the medial thigh lift.

Time: Depending on the excision pattern in the upper thigh crease, some perform closures in the frog-leg position, whereas others turn the patient to the prone position to close the most posterior portion.

Caveat: When combining procedures with vectors of pull that oppose each other, results will be compromised, leaving behind loose skin.

Debulking Liposuction

When planning for the best results, consider debulking liposuction during the first stage. If on examination, it is noted that there is some tissue deflation but still significant adiposity, then the patient may benefit from liposuction to debulk the area before the excision. Debulking liposuction is most commonly beneficial in the upper arms and in the medial thighs. By performing the liposuction and allowing time for the tissue to deflate and skin to retract, the best aesthetic result can be achieved when performing the skin excision. When performing liposuction at the time of the excision, the amount should be more judicious because there will be greater swelling and likely return of some tissue laxity.

Time: As long as the areas of liposuction do not require a position change, this can be done relatively quickly and added on to any of the above stages.

Caveat: When performing liposuction at the time of the excision, the amount should be more judicious because there will be greater swelling and likely return of some tissue laxity.

SUMMARY

The demand for body contouring surgery is increasing, and plastic surgeons must understand how to properly evaluate the patient and plan and execute safe surgical procedures:

- Perform a comprehensive medical workup and pay specific attention to weight history and nutritional status
- BMI greater than 30 is associated with increased postoperative complications
- Outcomes are optimized when weight is stable for at least 3 months
- Perform a detailed physical examination. Evaluate for skin excess and elasticity and distinguish between intraperitoneal and subcutaneous fat
- Patients who want multiple areas addressed will require staging
- Understanding which procedures are best paired to produce the best aesthetic outcome
- Consider patient's goals and try to address their top priorities is the first operation

REFERENCES

1. Matory WE Jr, O'Sullivan J, Fudem G, et al. Abdominal surgery in patients with severe morbid obesity. Plast Reconstr Surg 1994;94:976–87.
2. Vastine VL, Morgan RF, Williams GS, et al. Wound Complications of abdominoplasty in obese patients. Ann Plast Surg 1999;42:34–9.
3. Arthurs ZM, CUadrado D, Sohn V, et al. Post-bariatric panniculectomy body mass index impacts the complication profile. Am J Surg 2007;193:567–70.
4. Almutairi K, Gusenoff JA, Rubin JP. Body contouring. Plast Reconstr Surg 2016;137:586e–602e.
5. Capla J, Rubin JP. Staging and combining procedures. In: Rubin JP, editor. Body contouring and liposuction. Saunders; 2013. p. 593–603.
6. Rios LM, Khosla RK. Body contouring in the massive-weight-loss patient. In: Janis JE, editor. Essentials of plastic surgery. Thieme; 2017. p. 1285–99.
7. Bossert RP, Rubin JP. Evaluation of the weight loss patient presenting for plastic surgery consultation. Plast Reconstr Surg 2012;130:1361–9.

8. Oppikofer C, Law B, Schwappach D. The role of checklists and human factors for improved patient safety in plastic surgery. Plast Reconstr Surg 2017; 140:812e–7e.

9. Hardy KL, Davis KE, Constantine RS, et al. The impact of operative time on complications after plastic surgery: a multivariate regression analysis of 1753 cases. Aesthet Surg J 2014;34:614–22.

10. Czerniak S, Gusenoff JA, Rubin JP. Discussion: safety of outpatient circumferential body lift evidence from 42 consecutive cases. Plast Reconstr Surg 2017;139:1363–4.

Patient-Reported Outcome Measures: BODY-Q

Lotte Poulsen, MD[a], Giancarlo McEvenue, MD[b], Anne Klassen, DPhil[c],
Maarten Hoogbergen, MD, PhD[d], Jens Ahm Sorensen, MD, PhD[a],
Andrea Pusic, MD, PhD[e],*

KEYWORDS

- Bariatric surgery • Massive weight loss • Body contouring • Aesthetic surgery • Obesity
- Outcomes • Quality of life • BODY-Q

KEY POINTS

- Weight loss following lifestyle changes or bariatric surgery can result in functionally impairing excesses of skin.
- Surgical body contouring procedures have the potential to improve appearance and health-related quality of life.
- Patient-reported outcome measures (PROMs) are questionnaires designed to measure how patients function and feel from their point of view.
- The BODY-Q is a PROM designed to measure outcomes over the entire patient journey from the presurgery state (ie, obesity) to postsurgery after body contouring.
- The BODY-Q can be used to incorporate the patient perspective in massive weight loss and body contouring research, quality-improvement activities, and clinical practice.

INTRODUCTION

Body contouring encompasses a range of surgical procedures on different areas of the body and is one of the most rapidly growing areas within plastic surgery. According to the American Society for Aesthetic Plastic Surgery's 2016 statistics, the performance of lower body lifts has increased 360% since 1997 and arm lifts have increased 878% over the same time period.[1] The growth in body-contouring procedures parallels the increasing number of people undergoing bariatric surgery for morbid obesity, which in 2016 was estimated to be 216,000 patients in the United States.[2] Bariatric surgery not only results in weight loss but also improves or resolves a range of comorbid obesity-related health conditions. However, at the end of the weight loss journey, many patients who undergo bariatric surgery are left with a huge amount of excess skin.[3] The

Disclosure: The qualitative portion of the BODY-Q study was supported by The Plastic Surgery Foundation. The international field-test was funded by a grant from the Canadian Institutes for Health Research (CIHR). The BODY-Q is owned by McMaster University and Memorial Sloan-Kettering Cancer Center. A. Klassen and A. Pusic are co-developers of the BODY-Q and, as such, could potentially receive a share of any license revenues as royalties based on their institutions inventor sharing policy. Dr A. Pusic received support through the NIH/NCI Cancer Center Support Grant P30 CA008748. The BODY-Q study was funded by a National Endowment from the Plastic Surgery Foundation and an operating grant from the Canadian Institutes for Health Research. In addition, A. Klassen held a CIHR Mid-Career Award in Women's Health.
[a] Department of Plastic Surgery, Odense University Hospital, J. B. Winsløws Vej 4, Odense 5000, Denmark; [b] The McLean Clinic, Mississauga, Canada; [c] Department of Pediatrics, McMaster University, Hamilton, Canada; [d] Department of Plastic and Reconstructive Surgery, Catharina Hospital, Michelangelolaan 2, 5623 EJ Eindhoven, Netherlands; [e] Department of Plastic and Reconstructive Surgery, Brigham and Women's Hospital, Harvard University, 75 Francis Street, Boston, MA 02115, USA
* Corresponding author.
E-mail address: apusic@bwh.harvard.edu

Clin Plastic Surg 46 (2019) 15–24
https://doi.org/10.1016/j.cps.2018.08.003

areas commonly affected by skin redundancy are circumferentially at the waist, upper thighs, upper arms, upper chest, and face. This excess skin is not only cosmetically unsightly but is also detrimental to body image and physical, psychological, and social function, that is, health-related quality of life (HR-QOL).[4,5] Even though this excess skin has been shown to be detrimental to HR-QOL, only one-quarter of patients who undergo bariatric surgery also undergo body contouring surgery mainly because of the high cost of surgery, which is often considered by health care payers to be cosmetic rather than reconstructive in nature.[5]

Traditional surgical outcome measures for bariatric and body contouring have focused on decreasing complication rates and improving aesthetic scores.[6–8] Most ratings of aesthetic outcomes in research to date have been limited to objective surgeon ratings.[9] These traditional outcomes do not offer a complete assessment of outcomes as they fail to take into account the patient's perspective. A full picture of the impact of bariatric and body contouring surgery should include measures of how patients function and feel at the start of their weight loss journey, and their health care experiences, and how these measures change over time as they lose weight.[10] To provide this full picture from the patients' perspective, a new questionnaire was needed.

Patient-Reported Outcomes

Patient-reported outcomes (PROs) represent patients' assessments of how they function or feel from their perspective without interference by clinicians or any other intermediary. A patient-reported outcome measure (PROM) is a questionnaire developed to measure a PRO. In recent years, PROMs have been increasingly used in both clinical practice and research, either instead of or as supplement to traditional objective measures. The Center for Devices and Radiological Health describes a greater than 500% increase in the use of PROMs over a 6-year period.[11] The use of a PROM in bariatric and body contouring is important because the goals of treatment include improvement of HR-QOL and appearance, outcomes best assessed by patients.[5,12] To ensure that PROMs used in bariatric and body contouring provide meaningful measurement, it is important that they are rigorously developed, psychometrically sound, and clinically meaningful. Systematic reviews have pointed out that PROMs used in bariatric surgery research to date have often been generic (eg, 36-Item Short Form Health Survey) and miss certain key concepts important

to patients undergoing weight loss. The use of condition-specific PROMs can overcome the limitations of such generic scales by asking relevant questions about outcomes that matter to patients.[13]

THE BODY-Q

The BODY-Q[10,14,15] is a PROM developed to measure outcomes that matter to patients undergoing weight loss due to lifestyle changes or bariatric surgery and/or body contouring surgery. The authors' team previously described the need for a PROM specifically for this patient population.[3,16] To develop a PROM that covers issues that are relevant to both weight loss and body contouring surgery required a mixed-methods approach that involves extensive qualitative research to identify concerns that are common across patient groups, followed by advanced statistical techniques to identify any items biased by those characteristics. The development of the BODY-Q followed internationally recommended guidelines to maximize both the clinical meaning and scientific quality of each scale. The authors' approach to the development of the BODY-Q engaged patients and clinicians in the qualitative phase as experts whose input was critical to the design of the content of each scale. The authors aimed to ensure that the BODY-Q was valid and reliable for use in health research as well as in clinical care with individual patients. The authors used a 3-phased mixed-methods approach that they have previously published elsewhere (**Fig. 1**).[17] Each phase covers specific steps for item generation, item reduction, and psychometric evaluation.[18–23]

Briefly, in phase 1, qualitative methods were used to develop a conceptual framework and to generate a pool of items. These items were developed from a review of the literature and 63 patient interviews. The item pool was developed into scales, which were pilot tested with 22 patients and 9 clinical experts to clarify ambiguities in item wording, confirm appropriateness, and determine acceptability and completion time. In phase 2, the questionnaire was field tested in an international sample of 734 patients from Canada, the United States, and the United Kingdom. The questions that represented the best indicators of outcomes were retained based on their performance against a set of psychometric criteria using a modern item response theory approach called Rasch Measurement Theory (RMT) analysis.[24] In this approach, the qualitative phase was crucial because for each scale the data were used to design a set of items that together map out a construct on a clinical hierarchy. The

| PHASE | PURPOSE | COMPONENT | PRODUCT |

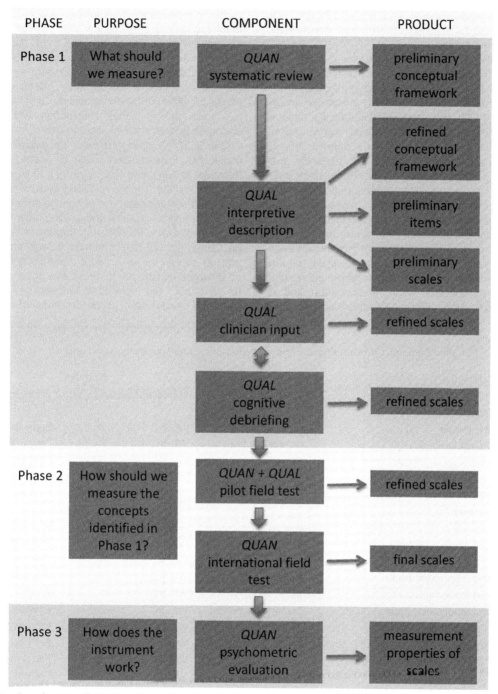

Fig. 1. Flow diagram illustrating the method for developing the BODY-Q. QUAN, quantitative study component; QUAL, qualitative study component.

RMT analysis confirmed that the data collected fit the Rasch model for each BODY-Q scale, providing a set of scales with linearised scores. In phase 3, the authors conducted a prospective study of 58 patients who were exploring or seeking bariatric surgery at the time of the BODY-Q field-test study. These patients were invited to complete the BODY-Q 2 years after bariatric surgery to assess the scales' ability to measure change. The mean percentage of total weight loss was 31%. Participants improved on BODY-Q scales measuring appearance, body image, and physical and social function with moderate to large effect sizes and standardized response means.

Table 1 shows characteristics for each BODY-Q scale. The HR-QOL domain consists of 5 different scales that cover physical, psychological, social and sexual function, and body image. To ensure that HR-QOL data are condition specific, patients are asked to answer all questions "with your body in mind." For the appearance domain, the 12 scales ask about satisfaction with the body, specifically different body parts (abdomen, back, inner thighs, hips and outer thighs, buttocks, upper arms, chest, and nipples). For excess skin, body contouring scars, and stretch marks, response options ask respondents to indicate how bothered they are from *not at all* to *extremely bothered*. The 4 scales designed to improve quality-of-care measure patient experience in terms information provided, doctor/surgeon, medical team, and office staff. All 21 BODY-Q scales were designed

to be independently functioning, which means that researchers or clinicians can choose from the full list of scales to use the ones that are most relevant to the research study or clinical scenario and thereby minimize respondent burden. For example, for a comparative effectiveness study of different abdominoplasty techniques, the scale asking about satisfaction with the abdomen is likely the key scale to use.

The BODY-Q does not have an overall total score, but instead each scale is scored from 0 (worse) to 100 (best). This approach to separate scores provides a more nuanced picture of patients and enables detection of change among patients starting at obesity and ending after body contouring. Some PROMs (eg, Impact of Weight on Quality of Life-Lite) consider it legitimate to add up scores for scales that measure a range of different constructs to provide a total score for HR-QOL (eg, physical function + self-esteem + sexual life + public distress and work).

Table 1
BODY-Q scales/checklist, number of items and intended body areas, patient group and time-point

Scale	Body Areas	Patient Group	Number of Items	Time Points
Health-related quality of life				
Body image	Overall	WL, BC	7	Pre/post
Physical function	Overall	WL, BC	7	Pre/post
Psychological function	Overall	WL, BC	10	Pre/post
Sexual function	Overall	WL, BC	5	Pre/post
Social function	Overall	WL, BC	10	Pre/post
Appearance				
Satisfaction with abdomen	Abdomen	WL, BC	7	Pre/post
Satisfaction with arms	Upper arms	WL, BC	7	Pre/post
Satisfaction with back	Back	WL, BC	4	Pre/post
Satisfaction with body	Body	WL, BC	10	Pre/post
Satisfaction with buttocks	Buttocks	WL, BC	5	Pre/post
Satisfaction with chest	Chest (only males)	WL, BC	10	Pre/post
Satisfaction with nipples	Nipples (only males)	WL, BC	5	Pre/post
Satisfaction with hips & outer thighs	Hip & outer thighs	WL, BC	5	Pre/post
Satisfaction with inner thighs	Inner thighs	WL, BC	4	Pre/post
Appraisal of excess skin	Excess skin	WL, BC	7	Pre/post
Appraisal of scars	Scars	BC	10	Post
Appraisal of stretch marks	Overall	WL, BC	10	Pre/post
Patient experience of care				
Satisfaction with doctor/surgeon	Overall	WL, BC	10	Post
Satisfaction with information	Overall	WL, BC	10	Post
Satisfaction with medical team	Overall	WL, BC	10	Post
Satisfaction with office staff	Overall	WL, BC	10	Post
Obesity-specific symptom checklist	Overall	WL	11	Pre/post

Abbreviations: BC, body contouring; WL, weight loss.

This approach to measurement, which is based on the classic test theory approach to scale development, is limited in that total scores can hide treatment effects, that is, when patients improve in some areas while deteriorating in others. An important strength of the BODY-Q is the use of a modern psychometric method, that is, RMT analysis.[24] The BODY-Q's ability to measure change over the entire patient journey (from obese to after body contouring surgery) is strengthened by the modern psychometric approach taken to develop the BODY-Q. This approach provides a set of unidimensional scales that have interval level measurement properties. Because of these measurement properties, the BODY-Q is an ideal PROM for use in both research and clinical practice settings with patients undergoing bariatric surgery and/or body contouring.

An advantage of the modular approach to scale development is that new scales can be added as a need for them is identified. The BODY-Q field-test study tested 18 independently functioning scales and an obesity-specific symptom checklist. Since then, the authors have developed and tested a new BODY-Q Stretch Marks Scale to measure patient perceptions of stretch marks anywhere on the body. This new 10-item scale was completed by 630 participants. The authors also developed the BODY-Q Chest Module composed of a 10-item chest and 5-item nipples appearance scale. This module was field tested in an international sample of 739 patients having gynecomastia, weight loss, and gender-affirming surgery[10,14,15,25,26] bringing the BODY-Q now has 21 independently functioning scales.

How to Get the BODY-Q

The BODY-Q is free to nonprofit users, including academics and clinicians. The BODY-Q was developed in English but has been translated into numerous languages (**Table 2**). The BODY-Q is distributed by Mapi Research Trust.[27] In order to obtain the relevant version of the BODY-Q, an online request and a BODY-Q licensing agreement must be filled out. For commercial use of the BODY-Q, a license agreement and a user fee is required. Please follow the link https://eprovide.mapi-trust.org/instruments/body-q#online_distribu-tion for more information. If the BODY-Q is not available in a specific language, permission is needed from Mapi Research Trust[27] to perform a translation.

Data Collection

When working with PROMs, it is essential that the information comes from the patients without interference by clinicians, caregivers, or anyone else. In the BODY-Q field test, study data were collected via paper and pencil as well as electronically using Research Electronic Data Capture (REDCap). REDCap is a secure Web application for building and managing online surveys and databases that is free to nonprofit organizations.[28] The authors' team has created REDCap template files that can be obtained on request after signing a license. Using an online application provides the opportunity to incorporate rate branching logic, so that individual patients are only asked to complete the scales relevant to them, which limits time and burden for both patients and clinicians.

International Use of the BODY-Q

The BODY-Q was originally developed in English and field tested in Canada, the United States, and the United Kingdom but is increasingly used worldwide. Currently BODY-Q scales have been translated into 9 languages for use in the following countries: Denmark, Finland, France, Germany, Italy, Netherlands, Norway, Poland, and Sweden (see **Table 2**).

Translation of the BODY-Q into Danish provides an example of the application of best-practice guidelines for translation and linguistic validation published by the International Society for Pharmacoeconomics and Outcomes Research and the World Health Organization. These guidelines aim to develop a conceptual translation rather than a literal translation.[29,30] Following rigorously developed guidelines will ensure the conceptual equivalence and thereby the possibility to compare BODY-Q scores from different countries. Briefly, the following 7 steps were taken: (1) 2 independent forward translations (target language as mother tongue and fluent in English) resulting in a harmonized translation; (2) backward translation (English mother tongue and fluent in target language); (3) comparison of the back-translated version with the original BODY-Q; (4) expert panel meeting with participation of all translators and specialists to determine if the translated version is clinically relevant from the clinician perspective; (5) cognitive patient interviews to determine if instructions, response options, and items are unambiguous, understandable, and relevant to the target group; (6) further cognitive interviews with patients whereby findings from the previous interviews were incorporated; (7) independent proof reading by 2 clinicians, leading to the final translated version of the BODY-Q. The translation and psychometric validation process is described in detail in other publications.[31,32] Once the Danish team had finalized the translation, they conducted a

Table 2
Overview of translated BODY-Q scales

Scale	Country (Language)								
	Denmark (Danish)	France (French)	Finland (Finnish)	Germany (German)	Italy (Italian)	Netherlands (Dutch)	Norway (Norwegian)	Poland (Polish)	Sweden (Swedish)
Health-related quality of life									
Body image	x	—	x	x	x	x	—	x	x
Physical function	x	x	x	x	x	x	—	x	x
Psychological function	x	—	x	x	x	x	—	x	x
Sexual function	x	x	x	x	x	x	x	x	x
Social function	x	x	x	x	x	x	—	x	x
Appearance									
Satisfaction with abdomen	x	—	x	x	x	x	—	x	x
Satisfaction with arms	x	—	x	x	x	x	—	x	x
Satisfaction with back	x	—	x	x	x	x	—	x	x
Satisfaction with body	x	x	x	x	x	x	—	x	x
Satisfaction with buttocks	x	—	x	x	x	x	—	x	x
Satisfaction with chest	x	—	x	—	x	x	—	x	x
Satisfaction with nipples	x	—	x	—	x	x	—	x	x
Satisfaction with hips & outer thighs	x	—	x	x	x	x	—	x	x

Satisfaction with inner thighs	×	—	×	×	×	×	×	×
Appraisal of excess skin	×	×	×	×	×	×	×	×
Appraisal of scars	×	×	×	×	×	×	×	×
Appraisal of stretch marks	×	—	—	×	×	×	—	×
Patient experience of care								
Satisfaction with doctor/ surgeon	×	—	×	×	×	×	×	×
Satisfaction with information	×	—	×	×	×	×	×	×
Satisfaction with medical team	×	—	×	×	×	×	×	×
Satisfaction with office staff	×	—	×	×	×	—	×	×
Obesity-specific symptom checklist	×	—	×	×	×	×	×	×

field-test study that included 495 patients. This team used RMT analysis to examine each scale's psychometric properties and showed that the BODY-Q was a reliable and valid PROM for use in Danish bariatric and body contouring programs.[32]

DISCUSSION

The BODY-Q is a clinically meaningful and scientifically sound PROM that can be used to measure outcomes in weight loss and/or body contouring surgery. In a recent systematic review of 24 PROMs, the BODY-Q was recommended as the most suitable quality-of-life measurement instrument for bariatric and body contouring due based on its strong psychometric properties.[33] The BODY-Q can play a role in patient care, including patient education about expected outcomes found to be most important to other patients undergoing the same procedures. The authors' previously published study found that patients who underwent bariatric surgery did not expect to have as much excess skin as they had or how the excess skin would make them look and feel. Conversely, patients who had bariatric surgery were not expecting to look as good as they did after body contouring, which was described as a huge benefit (psychological and socially) and a positive surprise.[13] The BODY-Q could also be used to provide health care payers with value-based metrics from the patient perspective. The BODY-Q experience and outcome scales, for example, could provide patient-centered information for quality-improvement purposes, similar to the use of the BREAST-Q Satisfaction with Information scale as a quality indicator by the Centers for Medicare and Medicaid Services (CMS).[34] BODY-Q scales are used by the Michigan Bariatric Surgery Collaborative (funded by the CMS) that to date has collected data on more than 4000 patients with ongoing long-term follow-up.[35] In the United Kingdom, the BODY-Q is used alongside BREAST-Q and FACE-Q scales in the Royal College of Surgeons national quality-improvement initiative for cosmetic procedures.[36] Specifically, the Satisfaction with Abdomen and Satisfaction with Body scales are used to evaluate outcomes for all patients undergoing an abdominoplasty and liposuction procedures. Finally, the BODY-Q provides a validated standardized measurement tool that can enable international research collaboration in outcomes research. Currently, researchers in several European countries are collecting and pooling BODY-Q data to build an evidence base for changes in appearance and HR-QOL in patients undergoing body contouring

following massive-weight-loss body contouring. The collection of large amounts of data for patients at varying points in their weight loss journey will allow for future benchmarking and normative data for interpretation of BODY-Q scores.[37,38]

Given advances in technology, PRO data can now be collected over the Internet or on a smart device with data transmitted directly into the electronic health records. Future directions for the BODY-Q include the collection and use of data in clinical practice. When used in clinical care, PROMs can provide patients with the opportunity to tell how they really feel and can help clinicians gain insight into a patient's symptoms and HR-QOL, which can help guide treatment decisions. A strength of the BODY-Q is the large number of independently functioning scales that measure outcomes important to patients. The authors previously reported that BODY-Q scales have high content validity as well as acceptability to patients who do not complain about the PROM length when asked to complete multiple scales but rather see it positively as an opportunity to provide insights into their experiences.[31] However, in some clinical and research settings there may be need for shorter assessments to reduce patient burden. The next stage of research for the BODY-Q is development of computer-adaptive testing (CAT). CAT is an innovative measurement approach, whereby the selection of questions (ie, items) is individualized for each patient.[39,40] This approach leads to a lower questionnaire burden with the same measurement precision.

SUMMARY

The BODY-Q provides the means to collect evidence-based outcomes data from the patient perspective. The authors encourage the health professionals involved in the care of (morbidly) obese patients to use this PROM. The information gained is needed to inform patient selection and education, comparative effectiveness research, and health care policy decisions.

REFERENCES

1. 2016 Cosmetic Surgery National Data Banks Statistics. The American Society for Aesthetic Plastic Surgery, 2016. Available at: https://www.surgery.org/sites/default/files/ASAPS-Stats2016.pdf. Accessed February 24, 2018.
2. Estimate of bariatric surgery numbers 2011-2016, American Society for Metabolic and Bariatric Surgery, 2016. Available at: https://asmbs.org/resources/estimate-of-bariatric-surgery-numbers. Accessed February 24, 2018.

3. Klassen AF, Cano SJ, Scott A, et al. Satisfaction and quality-of-life issues in body contouring surgery patients: a qualitative study. Obes Surg 2012;22(10): 1527–34.

4. Sarwer DB, Fabricatore AN. Psychiatric considerations of the massive weight loss patient. Clin Plast Surg 2008;35:10.

5. Poulsen L, Klassen A, Rose M, et al. Patient-reported outcomes in weight loss and body contouring surgery: a cross-sectional analysis using the BODY-Q. Plast Reconstr Surg 2017;140(3): 491–500.

6. Hurwitz DJ, Agha-Mohammadi S. Post-bariatric surgery breast reshaping: the spiral flap. Ann Plast Surg 2006;56:481–6.

7. Migliori F, Rosati C, D'Alessandro G, et al. Body contouring after biliopancreatic diversion. Obes Surg 2006;16:1638–44.

8. van Huizum MA, Roche NA, Hofer SO. Circular belt lipectomy: a retrospective follow-up study on perioperative complications and cosmetic outcome. Ann Plast Surg 2005;54:459–64.

9. McEvenue G, Xu F, Cai R, et al. Female-to-male gender affirming top surgery: a single surgeon's 15-year retrospective review and treatment algorithm. Aesthet Surg J 2017;38(1):49–57.

10. Klassen AF, Cano SJ, Scott A, et al. Assessing outcomes in body contouring. Clin Plast Surg 2014; 41(4):645–54.

11. Value and use of patient-reported outcomes (PROs) in assessing effects of medical devices. CDRH strategic priorities 2016-2017. Available at: https://www.fda.gov/downloads/AboutFDA/CentersOffices/OfficeofMedicalProductsandTobacco/CDRH/CDRHVisionandMission/UCM588576.pdf. Accessed February 12, 2018.

12. Poulsen L, Klassen A, Jhanwar S, et al. Patient expectations of bariatric and body contouring surgery. Plast Reconstr Surg Glob Open 2016;4(4):e694.

13. US food and drug administration clinical outcome assessment qualification program. FDA, 2015. Available at: http://www.fda.gov/Drugs/DevelopmentApprovalProcess/DrugDevelopmentToolsQualificationProgram/ucm284077.htm. Accessed February 12, 2018.

14. Klassen A, Cano SJ, Alderman A, et al. The BODY-Q: a patient-reported outcome instrument for weight loss and body contouring treatments. Plast Reconstr Surg Glob Open 2016;4(4):e679.

15. Klassen AF, Cano SJ, Kaur M, et al. Further psychometric validation of the BODY-Q: ability to detect change following bariatric surgery weight gain and loss. Health Qual Life Outcomes 2017;15(1):227.

16. Reavey PL, Klassen AF, Cano S, et al. Measuring quality-of-life and patient satisfaction after body contouring: a systematic review of patient-reported outcome measures. Aesthet Surg J 2011;31:807–13.

17. Wong Riff KW, Tsangaris E, Goodacre T, et al. International multiphase mixed methods study protocol to develop a cross-cultural patient-reported outcome instrument for children and young adults with cleft lip and/or palate (CLEFT-Q). BMJ Open 2017;7(1):e015467.

18. Lasch KE, Marquis P, Vigneux M, et al. PRO development: rigorous qualitative research as the crucial foundation. Qual Life Res 2010;19:1087–96.

19. Patrick DL, Burke LB, Gwaltney CJ, et al. Content validity-establishing and reporting the evidence in newly developed Patient-Reported Outcomes (PRO) instruments for medical product evaluation: ISPOR PRO good research practices task force report: part 1- eliciting concepts for a new PRO instrument. Value Health 2011;14:967–77.

20. Scientific Advisory Committee of the Medical Outcomes Trust. Assessing health status and quality of life instruments: attributes and review criteria. Qual Life Res 2002;11:193–205.

21. The COSMIN checklist. Available at: http://www.cosmin.nl/COSMIN%20checklist.html. Accessed February 12, 2018.

22. Mokkink LB, Terwee CB, Patrick DL, et al. The COSMIN study reached international consensus on taxonomy, terminology, and definitions of measurement properties for health-related patient-reported outcomes. J Clin Epidemiol 2010;63:737–45.

23. Mokkink LB, Terwee CB, Patrick DL, et al. The COSMIN checklist for assessing the methodological quality of studies on measurement properties of health status measurement instruments: an international Delphi study. Qual Life Res 2010;18: 539–49.

24. Rasch measurement theory. Available at: http://www.rasch.org/rmt/rmt74m.htm. Accessed February 10, 2018.

25. Poulsen L, Pusic A, Robson S, et al. The BODY-Q stretch marks scale: a development and validation study. Aesthet Surg J 2018;38(9):990–7.

26. Klassen AF, Kaur M, Poulsen L, et al. The BODY-Q chest module for adolescents boys, men and trans men who undergo masculinizing chest contouring surgery for weight loss, gynaecomastia, and gender dysphoria. Plast Reconstr Surg, in press.

27. Mapi Research Trust, ePROVIDE, online support for clinical outcome assessments. Available at: https://eprovide.mapi-trust.org/instruments/body-q#online_distribution. Accessed February 11, 2018.

28. REDCap. Available at: https://www.project-redcap.org. Accessed February 11, 2018.

29. Wild D, Grove A, Martin M, et al. Principles of good practice for the translation and cultural adaptation process for Patient-Reported Outcomes (PRO) measures: report of the ISPOR task force for translation and cultural adaptation. Value Health 2005;8(2): 94–104.

30. Process of translation and adaptation of instruments, World Health Organization. Available at: http://www.who.int/substance_abuse/research_tools/translation/en/. Accessed February 12, 2018.

31. Poulsen L, Rose M, Klassen A, et al. Danish translation and linguistic validation of the BODY-Q: a description of the process. Eur J Plast Surg 2017; 40(1):29–38.

32. Poulsen L, Klassen A, Rose M, et al. Psychometric validation of the BODY-Q in Danish patients undergoing weight loss and body contouring surgery. Plast Reconstr Surg Glob Open 2017;5(10):e1529.

33. de Vries CEE, Kalff MC, Prinsen CAC, et al. Recommendations on the most suitable quality-of-life measurement instruments for bariatric and body contouring surgery: a systematic review. Obes Rev 2018. [Epub ahead of print].

34. Centers for medicare & medicaid services, quality indicators. Available at: https://www.plasticsurgery.org/documents/medical-professionals/quality-resources/Measures- Included-in-the-2018-QCDR.pdf. Accessed March 11, 2018.

35. Michigan bariatric surgery collaborative. Available at: http://michiganbsc.org. Accessed March 16, 2018.

36. Royal College of Surgeons, patient reported outcome measures. Available at: https://www.rcseng.ac.uk/standards-and-research/standards-and-guidance/service-standards/cosmetic-surgery/clinical-quality-and-outcomes/patient-reported-outcome-measures/. Accessed March 11, 2018.

37. Mundy LR, Homa K, Klassen AF, et al. Normative data for interpreting the BREAST-Q: augmentation. Plast Reconstr Surg 2017;139(4):846–53.

38. Mundy LR, Homa K, Klassen AF, et al. Breast cancer and reconstruction: normative data for interpreting the BREAST-Q. Plast Reconstr Surg 2017;139(5):1046e–55e.

39. Cook KF, O'Malley KJ, Roddey TS. Dynamic assessment of health outcomes: time to let the CAT out of the bag? Health Serv Res 2005;40(5):1694–711.

40. Ware JE Jr, Kosinski M, Bjorner JB, et al. Applications of computerized adaptive testing (CAT) to the assessment of headache impact. Qual Life Res 2003;12(8):935–52.

Safety in Body Contouring to Avoid Complications

George Kokosis, MD, Devin Coon, MD, MSE*

KEYWORDS

- Body contouring • Safety • Abdominoplasty • Massive weight loss

KEY POINTS

- Comorbidities and body habitus make body contouring after massive weight loss challenging.
- Preoperatively the plastic surgeon needs to assess the clinical suitability of a patient to undergo surgery and manage expectations.
- Careful physical examination, photographic documentation, and standardized approach focusing on staging of the procedures and choosing the appropriate setting (outpatient vs inpatient) can be major determinants of outcomes.
- Smoking cessation, assessment of nutritional deficits, and evaluation of over-the-counter herbals consumption and their cessation are paramount.
- Prevention of hypothermia and appropriate positioning between supine, lateral decubitus, and prone positions need to be smooth and coordinated.

INTRODUCTION

According to the Centers for Disease Control and Prevention, in 2015 the prevalence of obesity (body mass index [BMI] >30 kg/m^2) was 36% among adults and 17% among youth.[1] Morbid obesity (BMI >40 kg/m^2) is also rising, with recorded prevalence of almost 7%. Obesity is associated with comorbidities, such as obstructive sleep apnea, type 2 diabetes mellitus, coronary artery disease, and stroke, all leading causes of preventable death.[2] Although a few patients can lose weight with dietary changes and exercise programs, the majority ultimately require weight loss surgery. Advances in surgical techniques and gaining of experience have pushed the limits of appropriateness of patients as surgical candidates and increased the rates of bariatric surgery.[3] The implications of bariatric surgery growth are significant because extensive data support improvement or resolution of obesity-associated comorbidities at a rate of 80%.[4]

Successful weight loss, however, creates a new challenge for patients, who face problems with excess skin and lipodystrophy, contour deformities, and physical challenges, such as intertrigo, fungal infections, ulcerations, and other hygiene issues. After the appropriate weight loss, more patients are now seeking body-contouring surgeries. Kitzinger and colleagues[5] in 2012 reported that 25% of women and 6% of men are pursuing postbariatric body-contouring surgery. It is imperative for plastic surgeons who perform this surgery to understand the challenges associated with this unique patient population. Poor outcomes can be linked to post–weight loss issues, such as residual nutritional deficiencies and chronic anemia as well as psychological burdens. The complications associated with body-contouring surgery in the weight loss patients are as high as 50% to 70%, most commonly in the form of minor wound complications like dehiscence and seroma formation.[6] The goal of this review is to highlight pearls that plastic surgeons can incorporate to minimize

Disclosure Statement: The authors have nothing to disclose.
Department of Plastic and Reconstructive Surgery, Johns Hopkins University, 601 North Caroline street, Baltimore, MD 21287, USA
* Corresponding author.
E-mail addresses: dcoon@jhmi.edu; theobc@gmail.com

Clin Plastic Surg 46 (2019) 25–32
https://doi.org/10.1016/j.cps.2018.08.004
0094-1298/19/© 2018 Elsevier Inc. All rights reserved.

these complications and maximize safety. A standardized approach that provides safe and successful care of these patients starts in the consultation room, with identifying all the preoperative needs and pertinent physiology; continues in the operating room, with appropriate preventative measures and state-of-the-art surgical technique; and addresses all postoperative needs with anticipatory planning.

THE PREOPERATIVE EVALUATION
Body Mass and Current Weight

A key variable that can affect outcomes is the BMI of the patient at the time of body contouring (**Box 1**). Starting weight prior to weight loss surgery is not the same across different patients; therefore, the final goal weight leading to the body-contouring procedures is also different but often still in the obese range of BMI greater than or equal to 30. There is evidence that residual obesity as evident by high BMI is associated with higher rates of complications, although there are conflicting results in the literature. Arthurs and colleagues[7] in their study showed that BMI greater than 25 multiplied the risk of postoperative complications by a factor of 3. Nemerofsky and colleagues[8] reported that BMI greater than 32 is associated with higher complication rates, although these results were not statistically significant. Other studies have reported similar outcomes between different BMI indices.[9]

The authors previously studied this effect in a prospective cohort of 449 patients who underwent 511 body-contouring procedures.[10] Maximum BMI and differences in BMI between weight loss

---

Box 1
Considerations during the preoperative evaluation

- Patients should have demonstrated stable weight for 3 months to 6 months.
- Patients must refrain from smoking for 2 weeks to 6 weeks prior to their surgery.
- Thorough physical examination and documentation (both in medical record and with the use of photographs) of findings, including prior scars, is paramount.
- Preoperative evaluation taking into consideration all comorbidities, nutritional deficits, and use of herbals
- Provide patients with detailed explanation of potential outcomes and detect possible divergence from their expectations.

---

and body-contouring surgery (ΔBMI) but not current BMI were correlated with increased complication rates among patients undergoing multiple body-contouring procedures in 1 stage. In the group of patients undergoing a single operation, maximum BMI and current BMI were associated with higher complication rates. A high BMI beyond 40 should be deemed challenging, and generally the authors only offer a body-contouring procedure to patients with an indication that poses risks to their health (eg, massive pannus or buried penis) who are unable to lose weight first, accepting the potentially higher risk in this patient cohort.

The authors' current belief is that ΔBMI is correlated with complications because it is a predictor of the magnitude of the surgery. Although elevated current BMI seems to increase the rate of wound complications and impairs the aesthetic result, if it is not excessively high, (eg, BMI >40) surgery can still be successful.

Weight Stability

To evaluate a patient for body-contouring surgery, there should ideally be a stable weight (within 5 kg of the target weight) for at least 3 months to 6 months.[11,12] A majority of plastic surgeons wait for 12 months to 18 months after the index bariatric operation before the body contouring takes place.[11,13]

Smoking

Patients who smoke are prone to exceedingly elevated complication rates, mainly skin necrosis and infection as well as wound dehiscence.[14,15] It may be the single greatest modifiable risk factor. Although not universally used, a urine cotinine test can be performed as a means of objective data on tobacco abstinence, because some patients may not be honest regarding nicotine use if they are aware that admitting smoking may lead to deferral of surgery.[15] The weakest area of evidence is regarding how long a period of nicotine cessation is necessary before perioperative risk normalizes; as a result, although some surgeons ask for 2 weeks to 3 weeks of cessation, some surgeons wait for at least 4 weeks[16] or even 3 months before they operate.[13]

Physical Examination

Evaluation and documentation of the deformities should be performed in a systematic fashion. There are classification systems that can facilitate this process.[17] History of skin rashes, breakdown, and prior infections needs to be documented. Skin excess and fascial laxity per body part need to be evaluated. Scars from prior operations, mainly the abdominal scars from the bariatric surgery or even the location of the port in the case of a gastric band, need to be documented and taken into consideration when planning the surgical approach so that no skin flap compromise results.[13] Photographic documentation is also important at this point because it helps demonstrate deformities and manage expectations.

Assess for Comorbidities

One of the most important determinants of postoperative complications is the medical and physical condition of the patient preoperatively. As discussed previously, many of the obesity-related comorbidities resolve after surgery but the exact status has to be evaluated prior to surgery. A primary care physician should provide preoperative medical risk stratification and clearance and, if deemed necessary, referral to medical subspecialists (eg, for cardiology evaluation if there is a concern for cardiac disease). These comorbidities should be at their most optimized state (eg, diabetes currently is as well-controlled as the endocrinologist expects it can be).

The American Society of Anesthesiologists (ASA) classification is a proved predictor of anesthetic and overall perioperative risk. Rohrich and colleagues[18] have suggested that central body lifts be limited to no higher than ASA class II. The family history as well as personal history of thrombus formation and postoperative complications is thoroughly delineated. The preoperative functional status of patients is also evaluated, because this often relates to how well they tolerate perioperative stress.

Use of Herbals

A unique perioperative challenge when evaluating postbariatric patients is the variable use of remedies and herbal supplements that become part of their postsurgical diet. The challenge with these remedies is 2-fold. Because they are not labeled as medications, patients often fail to report their use during interview. Many of them, however, may contain dangerous substances or interact with other prescription medications, such as the ones metabolized through the cytochrome P450 pathway, and cause perioperative side effects, such as bleeding, hypertension, or hypotension.[19] In the event they are using these medications, there is a consensus for stopping those at least 2 weeks prior to the operation.[20]

Assess for Nutritional Deficits

Another important aspect of preoperative evaluation for postbariatric patients seeking body-contouring surgery is their nutritional status. Postbariatric patients subject to malabsorptive procedures are prone to nutrient deficiencies, such as iron; folic acid; vitamins A, B_{12}, D, E, K, and C; zinc; and selenium. Additionally, due to food intolerance and significant change in taste, many of these patients end up developing protein malabsorption.[13,21,22] All these can lead to wound healing complications as well as other side effects. It is, therefore, wise to have the patients tested preoperatively for levels of electrolytes, vitamins, elements, and albumin/prealbumin. Any deficiency may warrant further nutritional evaluation and optimization prior to committing to a major body-contouring procedure. Many of these patients are placed on chronic supplementation of iron, folate, vitamin B_{12}, and others.

In particular, protein malnutrition is of paramount importance because patients usually overestimate their amount of caloric/protein intake and are unaware of an ongoing protein deficiency.[23] Adequate protein intake is essential for collagen synthesis and wound healing.

Psychosocial Issues/Expectations

Recognizing the unique psychosocial issues surrounding the postbariatric patient is a key element to deciding if the plastic surgeon will perform a body-contouring operation as well as the exact approach to setting expectations preoperatively. Approximately 40% of these patients have an active diagnosis of a psychiatric disorder and are on a medical regimen (mostly antidepressants) at the time of the consultation with the plastic surgeon.[24] This is not surprising if the association of binge-eating, obesity, and personality or mood disorders is understood. Active diagnosis of a psychiatric disorder should not be a contraindication to performing body contouring as long as a patient is well optimized. The plastic surgeon, however, should have a low threshold for postponing the procedure until a formal psychiatric consult is done if the surgeon believes that the patient is not optimized.[10,25] Additionally, body dysmorphic disorder is more prevalent in this population, with rates as high as 15%.[26] This leads to dissatisfaction after body contouring regardless of the aesthetic result. The plastic surgeon needs to identify all these risk factors and consider appropriately before any procedure is performed. In an effort to set the appropriate expectations, pictures of other patients who underwent body contouring with preprocedure and postprocedure captions can be helpful. Patients need to understand that they are exchanging the excess skin for long scars and potential complications.[19] A thorough discussion about the potential complications and the recovery plan in the early postoperative period sets an appropriate tone.

PREPARING FOR THE OPERATION
Plan a Staged Approach

Massive weight loss patients often require correction of multiple deformities from head to toe. It is known that increased duration of any procedure is directly linked to postoperative complications as the amount of anesthesia, blood loss, and fluid shift increases.[27] It is, therefore, imperative to stage the interventions and minimize the physiologic stress that is associated with increased operative time. Although it is common to stage body contouring, the exact number of stages and the type of procedures per stage varies between surgeons. The ultimate decision is based on several factors and is a mutual decision between the plastic surgeon and the patient.[14] These are usually a patient's main complaints: preoperative functional status and morbidity profile, the surgeon's experience and the level of assistance provided, and the financial burden associated. Coon and colleagues[28] suggested that when planning the staging, the surgical team should avoid opposing vectors, and procedures should take place in a setting with at least the option of inpatient admission, usually resulting in 2 to 3 stages for total body reshaping. The authors commonly combine a lower body–contouring procedure (ie, abdominoplasty) with an upper body–contouring procedure (ie, mastopexy). The authors try to avoid performing circumferential lower body lift and vertical thigh lift simultaneously because recovery from this combination is challenging.[14] Other investigators also report minimizing the procedures such that no stage lasts longer than 6 hours to 7 hours and each stage takes place at 3-month intervals.[29]

Outpatient Versus Inpatient Facility

Many postbariatric patients do not ultimately undergo body-contouring procedures due to the cost that is associated with these. One of the major determinants of the overall cost is whether the procedure takes place in an outpatient setting versus an inpatient setting, with the latter adding significant cost.[30] There is a growing body of literature supporting that performing traditionally major body-contouring procedures (such as circumferential lipectomy) in the outpatient setting is as safe as inpatient counterparts, while minimizing the cost and increasing access to this type of care. Which procedures and how many may be safely combined vary based on the patient, surgeon experience, and size of the operative

team. As long as the outpatient facility is appropriately equipped and meets the criteria of American Society of Plastic Surgeons guidelines, these procedures can be performed at an outpatient basis without compromising patient care (**Box 2**).

THE DAY OF SURGERY AND IN THE OPERATING ROOM
The Staff

It is important to approach these procedures as a team given the challenges that are associated with this patient population. The presence of an experienced anesthesiologist fully aware of a patient's comorbidities who is in control of all intraoperative variables, especially appropriate glycemic control, is valuable. Circulating nursing staff who can follow a standardized approach from the moment patients are in the preoperative holding area, when ready to undergo sterile prepping while awake positioning, and until they leave the perioperative area minimize any potential mistakes. Lastly, the leading surgeon should stage the procedures according to experience and the size of the surgical team to avoid excessive case duration.[11]

Perioperative Pain Control

It is vital to have good pain control for body contouring patients so they can mobilize as early as possible to minimize complications, such as deep vein thrombosis (venous thromboembolism [VTE]) or pulmonary embolism (PE), atelectasis, and pneumonia. There has been an extensive discussion regarding the opioid epidemic in the United States.[31] Patients need to have adequate analgesia ensured while avoiding narcosis, especially in this patient population, who may have present or resolving obstructive apnea. Regional blocks either after mastopexy (intercostal block)

Box 2
Considerations when preparing for the procedure

- Plan a staged approach to minimize perioperative complications.
- Each stage is usually limited to 6 hours' to 8 hours' maximum duration and at 3-month intervals.
- Outpatient operations can be performed in an appropriately equipped outpatient facility without compromising patient care.
- Proper selection of the right surgical setting for a given patient and procedure is essential.

or after abdominoplasty (transversus abdominis plane block) can also help with perioperative pain control.[32,33]

Positioning

Postbariatric procedures are often very long and can involve multiple positional changes increasing risk of an injury.[25] This is one of the more common causes of litigation for these cases.[34–36] Injuries can either result from traction or compression and the operating room team needs to coordinate during patient positioning to avoid any of these adverse outcomes (**Box 3**). In the supine position, the arms, elbows, and heels are padded to minimize pressure. When patients are placed prone, care must be taken to secure the endotracheal tube and avoid dislodgement. Intraocular pressure can increase significantly during long cases and prone positioning, and cases of visual loss have been reported.[37,38] A reverse Trendelenburg position of 15° may off-load the pressure and protect the eyes along with standard lubrication and taping of the eyes.[11] When a patient is repositioned to lateral decubitus, adequate padding of the axilla needs to be ensured to avoid traction on the brachial plexus.[19]

Temperature

Hypothermia, defined as core body temperature below 36°C, can lead to a variety of intraoperative or postoperative events, namely cardiac events, coagulopathy and increased blood loss, wound dehiscence, infection, and seroma.[25,39] In addition to strong evidence in general surgery, the senior author has shown that temperatures below 36°C strongly increase complications in body contouring specifically.[25] It is, therefore, imperative to prevent hypothermia, especially in the body-contouring patient where there is a large surface area exposed for a prolonged period of time. The Rubin protocol from the University of Pittsburgh includes a forced-flow air warmer used in the preoperative area, warming blankets used during the case, and room temperature maintained at 21°C (70°F).[25] The fluids used, including the betadine preparation kit, are prewarmed.

Venous Thromboembolism

VTE represents one of the deadliest adverse events after surgery and is more prevalent in the bariatric population. Studies reveal a rate of VTE at the range of 1% to 9.3%.[8,40] Abdominoplasty had the highest death rate secondary to PE in an outpatient facility.[41] There is controversy over the exact protocol in VTE prophylaxis in this patient population. The lack of evidence has led to wide variety of practices among body-contouring plastic surgeons, ranging from early mobilization and sequential compression devices with no chemoprophylaxis to 1 dose of low-molecular-weight heparin (LMWH) 1 hour preoperatively and then twice daily until discharge.[8,18,42,43]

Most guidelines stem from guidelines for general surgery patients and the American College of Chest Physicians,[44] which recommends either low-dose unfractionated heparin 3 times a day or LMWH once daily for high-risk patients, and body-contouring patients fall into this category. Timing of heparin administration and additional modalities are still not well defined for this specific patient population. Wes and colleagues[45] performed a National Surgical Quality Improvement Program database analysis of 17,774 patients and found that age over 45 years, with a BMI above 35; undergoing body contouring of the trunk and rather than 2 separate regions in the body; and inpatient status represent a higher risk group. In the plastic surgery literature, the Caprini score has been studied and used for risk stratification, with patients with a score greater than 7 to 8 benefitting from chemoprophylaxis.[46] The authors typically screen all patients for a personal of family history of thromboembolic events.[47] All patients have sequential compression devices placed and LMWH the night of surgery.[25] Patients with an extremely large pannus requiring giant panniculectomy may have an inferior vena cava filter by the vascular surgery service.

Box 3
Considerations in the operating room

- A standardized approach (prepping and positioning) by a team of professionals minimizes the chances of perioperative error.
- Perioperative pain control increases patient satisfaction and decreases perioperative complications.
- Avoid hypothermia.
- Screen patients for coagulopathies.
- Use combined modalities for thromboembolism prophylaxis, including sequential compression devices and chemoprophylaxis postoperatively.
- Use of drains, quilting sutures, and fibrin glue can decrease seroma rates.
- Meticulous dissection above nodal basins minimizes the incidence of lymphedema.

Prevention of Infection, Hematoma, Seroma, Skin Necrosis, and Lymphedema

The use of antibiotics within 30 minutes prior to the operation and redosing every 4 hours is accepted as a means of infection prevention.[48] Many prescribe antibiotics until drains are removed, although there are no good data on this practice. Meticulous hemostasis is key and clips should be placed on large-caliber vessels.

A variety of alternatives to drains have been used. There are several large series of progressive tension sutures showing they can decrease seroma rates.[49] Fibrin glue can also be used, although it seems there is no additive effect.[50]

Skin necrosis can be prevented if tension across the skin edges is limited and thus precise preoperative markings are of paramount importance with intraoperative confirmation using towel clips and the pinch test before resection. Following Lockwood's[51] concept of anchor lines, using the superficial fascial system for suspension results in more accurate and predictable results. Meticulous dissection above nodal basins when nearby, especially in the thighs and groins, can minimize the incidence of lymphedema.[52]

THE POSTOPERATIVE PERIOD

A uniform approach that engages the team and the patient is required to minimize preventative complications after body contouring. As discussed previously, drains should remain in place either for 10 days to 14 days or until the output is minimal. Early ambulation is a key component of VTE prophylaxis with chemoprophylaxis while an inpatient. Minor wound complications are common and are managed expectantly with local wound care and light débridement.

Garments or compression dressings are used to reduce swelling; caution needs to be focused, however, on avoidance of extreme pressure that compromises breathing or causes skin necrosis if pressure is applied against drains. Patients are encouraged to increase their protein intake in the early postoperative period (**Box 4**). Because appetite is generally decreased after surgery, supplements and even a nutritionist consultation can add benefit.

SUMMARY

Postbariatric body-contouring procedures are growing in popularity and patients can embark on a journey that offers them a second chance for a healthy, confident lifestyle, often resulting in some of the most grateful plastic surgery patients. It is important, however, to not underestimate the

---

> **Box 4**
> **Considerations in the early postoperative period**
>
> - Apply compression garments.
> - Mobilize patients early.
> - Encourage adequate intake to facilitate wound healing.
> - Drains need to be left for until low output is recorded.

---

magnitude of these procedures and challenges unique to this patient population. Prevention is the single most important factor in managing complications. A strategic approach starts from the consultation and appropriate patient selection with management of expectations. A team approach with safety protocols in the operating room ensures an optimal result, and close follow-up in the early postoperative period with clear instructions minimizes the incidence of complications and maximizes patient satisfaction.

REFERENCES

1. Cynthia L, Ogden PD, Margaret D, et al. Prevalence of obesity among adults and youth: United States, 2011-2014. 2015 edition. Hyattsville (MD): NCHS Data Brief; 2015.
2. Available at: https://www.cdc.gov/obesity/data/adult.html. Accessed February 17, 2018.
3. Daniel Guerron A, Portenier DD. Patient selection and surgical management of high-risk patients with morbid obesity. Surg Clin North Am 2016; 96:743.
4. Hng KN, Ang YS. Overview of bariatric surgery for the physician. Clin Med (Lond) 2012;12:435.
5. Kitzinger HB, Abayev S, Pittermann A. The prevalence of body contouring surgery after gastric bypass surgery. Obes Surg 2012;22(1):8–12.
6. Kitzinger HB, Cakl T, Wenger R, et al. Prospective study on complications following a lower body lift after massive weight loss. J Plast Reconstr Aesthet Surg 2013;66:231.
7. Arthurs ZM, Cuadrado D, Sohn V, et al. Post-bariatric panniculectomy: pre-panniculectomy body mass index impacts the complication profile. Am J Surg 2007;193:567.
8. Nemerofsky RB, Oliak DA, Capella JF. Body lift: an account of 200 consecutive cases in the massive weight loss patient. Plast Reconstr Surg 2006; 117:414.
9. Shermak MA, Chang D, Magnuson TH, et al. An outcomes analysis of patients undergoing body contouring surgery after massive weight loss. Plast Reconstr Surg 2006;118:1026.

10. Coon D, Gusenoff JA, Kannan N, et al. Body mass and surgical complications in the postbariatric reconstructive patient: analysis of 511 cases. Ann Surg 2009;249:397.

11. Colwell AS, Borud LJ. Optimization of patient safety in postbariatric body contouring: a current review. Aesthet Surg J 2008;28:437.

12. Hurwitz DJ. Single-staged total body lift after massive weight loss. Ann Plast Surg 2004;52:435.

13. Herman CK, Hoschander AS, Wong A. Post-bariatric body contouring. Aesthet Surg J 2015;35:672.

14. Almutairi K, Gusenoff JA, Rubin JP. Body contouring. Plast Reconstr Surg 2016;137:586e.

15. Coon D, Tuffaha S, Christensen J, et al. Plastic surgery and smoking: a prospective analysis of incidence, compliance, and complications. Plast Reconstr Surg 2013;131:385.

16. Krueger JK, Rohrich RJ. Clearing the smoke: the scientific rationale for tobacco abstention with plastic surgery. Plast Reconstr Surg 2001;108:1063.

17. Song AY, Jean RD, Hurwitz DJ, et al. A classification of contour deformities after bariatric weight loss: the Pittsburgh Rating Scale. Plast Reconstr Surg 2005;116:1535.

18. Rohrich RJ, Gosman AA, Conrad MH, et al. Simplifying circumferential body contouring: the central body lift evolution. Plast Reconstr Surg 2006;118:525.

19. Shermak MA. Pearls and perils of caring for the postbariatric body contouring patient. Plast Reconstr Surg 2012;130:585e.

20. Byard RW. A review of the potential forensic significance of traditional herbal medicines. J Forensic Sci 2010;55:89.

21. Heber D, Greenway FL, Kaplan LM, et al. Endocrine and nutritional management of the postbariatric surgery patient: an Endocrine Society Clinical Practice Guideline. J Clin Endocrinol Metab 2010;95:4823.

22. Faintuch J, Matsuda M, Cruz ME. Severe protein-calorie malnutrition after bariatric procedures. Obes Surg 2004;14:175.

23. Naghshineh N, O'Brien Coon D, McTigue K, et al. Nutritional assessment of bariatric surgery patients presenting for plastic surgery: a prospective analysis. Plast Reconstr Surg 2010;126:602.

24. Mitchell JE, Selzer F, Kalarchian MA. Psychopathology before surgery in the longitudinal assessment of bariatric surgery-3 (LABS-3) psychosocial study. Surg Obes Relat Dis 2012;8:533.

25. Michaels JT, Coon D, Rubin JP. Complications in postbariatric body contouring: strategies for assessment and prevention. Plast Reconstr Surg 2011;127:1352.

26. Crerand CE, Franklin ME, Sarwer DB. Body dysmorphic disorder and cosmetic surgery. Plast Reconstr Surg 2006;118:167e.

27. Procter LD, Davenport DL, Bernard AC, et al. General surgical operative duration is associated with increased risk-adjusted infectious complication rates and length of hospital stay. J Am Coll Surg 2010;210:60.

28. Coon D, Michaels Jt, Gusenoff JA, et al. Multiple procedures and staging in the massive weight loss population. Plast Reconstr Surg 2010;125:691.

29. Kenkel JM, Aly A, Capella J, et al. Body contouring surgery after massive weight loss "Examination of the Massive Weight Loss Patient and Staging Considerations". Plast Reconstr Surg 2006;117(1S):22S–30S.

30. Azin A, Zhou C, Jackson T, et al. Body contouring surgery after bariatric surgery: a study of cost as a barrier and impact on psychological well-being. Plast Reconstr Surg 2014;133:776e.

31. Geerts WH, Pineo GF, Heit JA, et al. Prevention of venous thromboembolism: the Seventh ACCP Conference on Antithrombotic and Thrombolytic Therapy. Chest 2004;126:338S.

32. Shah A, Rowlands M, Krishnan N, et al. Thoracic Intercostal nerve blocks reduce opioid consumption and length of stay in patients undergoing implant-based breast reconstruction. Plast Reconstr Surg 2015;136:584e.

33. Araco A, Pooney J, Araco F, et al. Transversus abdominis plane block reduces the analgesic requirements after abdominoplasty with flank liposuction. Ann Plast Surg 2010;65:385.

34. Shermak M, Shoo B, Deune EG. Prone positioning precautions in plastic surgery. Plast Reconstr Surg 2006;117:1584.

35. Prielipp RC, Morell RC, Butterworth J. Ulnar nerve injury and perioperative arm positioning. Anesthesiol Clin North America 2002;20:589.

36. Stewart JD, Shantz SH. Perioperative ulnar neuropathies: a medicolegal review. Can J Neurol Sci 2003;30:15.

37. Cheng MA, Todorov A, Tempelhoff R, et al. The effect of prone positioning on intraocular pressure in anesthetized patients. Anesthesiology 2001;95:1351.

38. Rupp-Montpetit K, Moody ML. Visual loss as a complication of non-ophthalmic surgery: a review of the literature. Insight 2005;30:10.

39. Coon D, Michaels Jt, Gusenoff JA, et al. Hypothermia and complications in postbariatric body contouring. Plast Reconstr Surg 2012;130:443.

40. Hatef DA, Kenkel JM, Nguyen MQ, et al. Thromboembolic risk assessment and the efficacy of enoxaparin prophylaxis in excisional body contouring surgery. Plast Reconstr Surg 2008;122:269.

41. Keyes GR, Singer R, Iverson RE, et al. Mortality in outpatient surgery. Plast Reconstr Surg 2008;122:245.

42. Aly AS, Cram AE, Chao M, et al. Belt lipectomy for circumferential truncal excess: the University of Iowa experience. Plast Reconstr Surg 2003;111:398.

43. Colwell AS, Borud LJ. Autologous gluteal augmentation after massive weight loss: aesthetic analysis and role of the superior gluteal artery perforator flap. Plast Reconstr Surg 2007;119:345.

44. Douketis JD, Berger PB, Dunn AS, et al. The perioperative management of antithrombotic therapy: American College of chest physicians evidence-based clinical practice guidelines (8th Edition). Chest 2008;133:299S.

45. Wes AM, Wink JD, Kovach SJ, et al. Venous thromboembolism in body contouring: an analysis of 17,774 patients from the National Surgical Quality Improvement databases. Plast Reconstr Surg 2015;135:972e.

46. Pannucci CJ, Swistun L, MacDonald JK, et al. Individualized venous thromboembolism risk stratification using the 2005 caprini score to identify the benefits and harms of chemoprophylaxis in surgical patients: a meta-analysis. Ann Surg 2017;265:1094.

47. Friedman T, O'Brien Coon D, Michaels JV, et al. Hereditary coagulopathies: practical diagnosis and management for the plastic surgeon. Plast Reconstr Surg 2010;125(5):1544–52.

48. Webb AL, Flagg RL, Fink AS. Reducing surgical site infections through a multidisciplinary computerized process for preoperative prophylactic antibiotic administration. Am J Surg 2006;192:663.

49. Pollock H, Pollock T. Progressive tension sutures: a technique to reduce local complications in abdominoplasty. Plast Reconstr Surg 2000;105:2583.

50. Bercial ME, Sabino Neto M, Calil JA, et al. Suction drains, quilting sutures, and fibrin sealant in the prevention of seroma formation in abdominoplasty: which is the best strategy? Aesthetic Plast Surg 2012;36:370.

51. Lockwood TE. Superficial fascial system (SFS) of the trunk and extremities: a new concept. Plast Reconstr Surg 1991;87:1009.

52. Michaels Jt, Coon D, Rubin JP. Complications in postbariatric body contouring: postoperative management and treatment. Plast Reconstr Surg 2011; 127:1693.

Pain Management and Body Contouring

Amanda Norwich, MD, Deepak Narayan, FRCS (Eng, Edin)*

KEYWORDS

- Postoperative pain • Preoperative pain • Pain control • Multimodal pain control
- Body contouring pain • Abdominoplasty pain • Breast augmentation pain • Mastopexy pain

KEY POINTS

- There are many effective alternatives to pain control for body contouring procedures, including prolonged or temporary local anesthetic and multimodal pain control.
- All approaches do not necessarily negate the need for opiate medications but aim to decrease their consumption.
- Nonopiate medications can be synergistic with other types of nonopiates as well as opiate medications.
- Studies show mixed results of the effect of nonsteroidal anti-inflammatory drug administration on postoperative bleeding.
- Prolonged local anesthesia is particularly effective in abdominoplasty, belt lipectomy, and breast augmentation procedures.

INTRODUCTION

The phrase *body contouring procedure* is a catchall term that includes mastopexy, breast augmentation, panniculectomy, abdominoplasty, liposuction, and lower body lift. It is well known that early ambulation is important in body contouring surgery, as in all surgical procedures. It limits hospitalization length of stay and decreases the incidence of complications, such as pulmonary embolism and atelectasis. Adequate pain control contributes greatly to patients' ability to ambulate. This is only one of the reasons pain control must be a priority for plastic surgeons. In this article, optimal medications and methods of analgesia are discussed. There have been many innovations in pain control beyond opiate medications, including prolonged administration of local anesthesia, regional blocks, and the multimodal approach, which emphasizes the use of nonopiate medications, such as nonsteroidal antiinflammatory drugs (NSAIDs). All approaches aim to decrease

oral or intravenous (IV) opiate use and, therefore, encourage faster return to normal bowel function and decreased risk of addiction. Considering the use of opiate medications is largely understood and already widely practiced, when discussing medications, the authors focus on nonopiates. This article is organized into general considerations in preoperative, intraoperative, and postoperative modalities and then focused further to discuss specific procedures. It should be noted the differentiation between preoperative, perioperative, and postoperative usage of medication is not always clear cut; therefore, there is some overlap in administration between sections.

PREOPERATIVE ANALGESIA

In this section regarding preoperative use of nonsteroidal medications, the authors mainly focus on oral cyclooxygenase-2 (COX-2) inhibitors. There has been controversy surrounding COX inhibitors because of concerns about postoperative

The authors have nothing to disclose.
Section of Plastic and Reconstructive Surgery, Department of Surgery, Yale School of Medicine, PO Box 208062, New Haven, CT 06520-8062, USA
* Corresponding author. 330 Cedar Street, 3rd Floor, New Haven, CT 06519.
E-mail address: deepak.narayan@yale.edu

Clin Plastic Surg 46 (2019) 33–39
https://doi.org/10.1016/j.cps.2018.08.005

gastrointestinal and surgical site bleeding. However, selective COX-2 inhibitors seem to have a lower risk of these complications. Other surgical specialties have successfully used celecoxib to decrease postoperative opiate use and hospital stay. In one study of colorectal surgery patients, preoperative celecoxib administration led to decreased hospital stay and decreased postoperative opiate use.[1] In obstetrics, preoperative rofecoxib (Vioxx) starting 1 hour before surgery decreased opiate use from 27% to 10%.[2] These findings were tempered by the recall of rofecoxib from the market in 2004 after studies showed it increased the risk of cardiovascular events. There has been some discussion recently about a small company named Tremeau Pharmaceuticals bringing rofecoxib back to market for severe hemophilia-related joint pain; however, this has not yet come to fruition.[3]

The void left behind by rofecoxib after its recall was filled by other COX-2 inhibitors, such as celecoxib (Celebrex), an effective antiinflammatory and analgesic. A study by Sun and colleagues[4] examined differences between placebo, postoperative, and preoperative administration of celecoxib to patients undergoing major plastic surgery. Procedures included breast augmentation and abdominoplasty with or without liposuction. Experimental groups received preoperative celecoxib with or without continuation of treatment in the first 3 postoperative days. Results showed opiate use in the first 3 postoperative days was significantly decreased in both experimental groups with the postoperative group consuming 18 mg, the preoperative group consuming 23 mg, and the control group consuming 68 mg of morphine within those three days. Average pain scores and return to bowel function were also significantly decreased. Number of days to return to daily activities of living was also decreased in experimental arms. Interestingly, there was no difference between the two intervention groups. Complication rates were comparable between control and experimental groups. It should be noted, and is discussed in other areas of this article, that patients undergoing body contouring procedures have often undergone weight loss surgery prior. In their discussion, Sun and colleagues[4] do not address the disadvantages of celecoxib after gastric bypass surgery. Although COX-2 inhibitors pose a lower risk of injury after gastric surgery, it is not the first choice of many bariatric surgeons.[5]

Acetaminophen is another powerful analgesic similar to NSAIDs with a partially understood mechanism of action that is used in perioperative care. In a study of 27 randomly selected participants undergoing abdominoplasty with rectus plication, patients were more likely to be discharged from the postanesthesia care unit (PACU) in the appropriate amount of time when given acetaminophen.[6] The control groups were given a standard preoperative pain regimen, whereas the experimental group had the standard regimen plus 1g IV acetaminophen before surgery. A goal time of 90 minutes from PACU to discharge was set. Seventy-three percent of patients receiving IV acetaminophen were discharged in the allotted amount of time versus 33% in the control arm. Researchers noted that the discrepancy was not always due to inadequate pain control; however, the substantial difference could not be ignored. There were no complications observed in patients given IV acetaminophen.

These results have been replicated in other procedures. In a double-blinded placebo-controlled trial by Moon and colleagues,[7] 76 women undergoing abdominal hysterectomy were randomized to patients receiving 2g IV acetaminophen or placebo 30 minutes preoperatively. Postoperative pain was treated with patient-controlled hydromorphone per protocol. The average 24-hour postoperative opiate use between groups was analyzed. Overall consumption of hydromorphone decreased by 30% in the experimental group. Postoperative nausea and vomiting substantially decreased as well. A significant drawback to the use of this medication is its cost compared with its oral counterpart. IV acetaminophen costs several-fold more than oral formulations. In one study, each vial of IV acetaminophen cost $10, whereas a 500-mg tablet costs $0.02.[8]

PERIOPERATIVE ANALGESIA

Perioperative analgesia is defined here as a combination of preoperative and postoperative administration of analgesics. Similar medications have been described for use purely preoperatively or postoperatively; however, it is important to note they can also be used for synergistic effect. One of the drugs that has been extensively studied in the perioperative context is pregabalin (Lyrica). In one placebo-controlled trial, pregabalin was added to a multimodal pain regimen including morphine, acetaminophen, and ibuprofen for 5 consecutive days after surgery.[9] Seventy-five milligrams were given the night before surgery, 1 hour before surgery, and continued twice a day for 4 days. No difference was observed in numerical movement-provoked pain scores 5 days after surgery or consumption of other pain medications. The investigators of this study noted the conflicting data on pregabalin use. A meta-analysis of studies using 300 mg or greater or less than 300 mg daily pregabalin administered preoperatively, perioperatively, or postoperatively showed mixed results.

The general consensus was a decrease in opiate use was noted, but there was no significant decrease in pain score at 24 hours. It was noted there may be advantages to using pregabalin; but it is difficult to standardize, as doses vary widely.[10]

However, there have been studies showing unequivocally favorable results with gabapentin. A meta-analysis performed in 2006 of perioperative gabapentin use in patients undergoing a variety of surgical procedures showed favorable results. Eighteen studies with a total of 1118 patients were included. Dosages ranged between 300 mg and 1200 mg daily. Most administered the first dose within hours of the operation, whereas fewer initiated therapy the day before surgery. Within the first 24 hours after surgery, total opiate consumption decreased by 35%.[11] Postoperative time at rest was decreased by 27% to 39%. Side effects included dizziness with a risk ratio of 1.4. Interestingly, the investigators of this article discuss postoperative pain in the context of central nervous system sensitization. Although the exact mechanism of gabapentin is unknown, it is related to decreased release of excitatory neurotransmitters, such as glutamate, substance P, and noradrenaline. This finding could account for its effectiveness as a pain modulator.

INTRAOPERATIVE ANALGESIA

The authors note at this time there is a paucity of data on parenteral intraoperative analgesia use. Local intraoperative analgesia is discussed in the procedure-specific section. With that said, one study found a difference between propofol and thiopentone. The study included 4173 patients and showed an 18% reduction in postoperative retching, nausea, and vomiting in patients in whom propofol was administered.[12] As postoperative nausea and vomiting may lead to seroma, clot release, hematoma, or dehiscence of suture lines, its prevention has a significant impact on patient outcomes.

Additionally, a local anesthetic not extensively discussed in further sections, but accepted widely as an effective analgesic, is liposomal bupivacaine (Exparel). This trademark multivesicular liposomal delivery system allows the bupivacaine to be encapsulated allowing delivery of the molecule in its unaltered state. Lipid membranes surround multiple aqueous chambers, which resorb into the body; the bupivacaine is slowly released over time. It has been shown liposomal bupivacaine can last up to 96 hours after injection. There are 2 peaks of efficacy, the first being at 0 to 2 hours and the second being at approximately 36 hours.[13] The maximum safe dose is 266 mg or 20 mL of a 1.3% solution. In a retrospective study of 64 female patients who underwent abdominoplasty with rectus plication, a liposomal bupivacaine solution was injected to select nerves supplying the abdominal wall. Surgeons injected deep to scarpa's fascia at the base of the flap, then laterally toward the external oblique fascia. Injections just deep to the fascial plication and in the pararectus space were also performed. The lateral and anterior cutaneous branches of the intercostal nerves, ilioinguinal nerve, and anterior cutaneous branch of the iliohypogastric nerve were targeted (**Fig. 1**). The average amount of opiate medication used, pain scores, and time to normal activity were compared with patients used in a previous study in which patients whereby patients received analgesia with pain pumps. Patients in the new trial decreased their use of postoperative pain pills to 14 from 16.8 at the time of their first postoperative visit. The authors' hypothesis is the directed nerve block with liposomal bupivacaine is more effective than bathing the nerves with local anesthetic, which is free to move and rest in pockets of the incision depriving other areas of pain relief. It was noted patients in this study underwent other, unidentified procedures ranging in severity.[13]

In a systemic review of liposomal bupivacaine used in plastic surgery procedures, a total of 8 articles were reviews, including 405 patients who underwent procedures, including breast

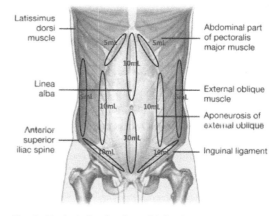

Fig. 1. Typical distribution of injections. A total injection volume of 80 mL (20 mL liposomal bupivacaine, 60 mL normal saline) is distributed over the abdominal wall for field block. (*Modified from* Drake, Richard Gray's Basic Anatomy, Second Edition. © 2017. Elsevier; with permission.)

reconstruction, breast augmentation, mammo-plasty, abdominal wall reconstruction, mastectomy, and abdominoplasty.[14] Liposomal bupivacaine was found to have adequate tolerability and safety as well as comparable or improved efficacy compared with traditional pain management. Studies reported high patient satisfaction, reduced opioid analge-sics, and decreased time to discharge. This article in particular suggested a standardized enhanced recovery after surgery protocol using liposomal bupivacaine. The investigators also note the versa-tility of liposomal bupivacaine, as it was used in a variety of procedures.

POSTOPERATIVE ANALGESIA

Management of acute postoperative pain while limiting opiate consumption is the goal of any sur-gical procedure. In addition to preoperative and intraoperative nonopiate medication administra-tion, as expected the postoperative regimen is very important. In this section, both medications and local analgesia techniques are discussed. As discussed above, paracetamol (acetaminophen) is a centrally acting analgesic and antipyretic used widely for pain control in surgical patients. A systematic review of studies looking at paracet-amol and NSAIDs showed the combination of paracetamol, a COX-2 inhibitor, and an NSAID decreased postoperative morphine consumption. However, it was difficult to distinguish between these 3 agents. Of note, when combined with an NSAID, paracetamol had increased efficacy. Addi-tionally, IV paracetamol is safe in the event pa-tients are allergic or unable to take NSAIDs, such as those patients with a peptic ulcer or asthma. A noted disadvantage of this regimen is the risk of hepatotoxicity with doses more than 4000 mg daily and its lack of efficacy in peripheral pain pathways. Specifically pertinent to surgical pa-tients is postoperative bleeding. In the same sys-tematic review, patients treated with NSAIDs experienced a 2.4% incidence of bleeding compared with 0.4% in controls.[15] Along these lines, a meta-analysis of ketorolac, a potent IV COX-1 inhibitor, showed no significant increase in postoperative bleeding when compared with control. The length of treatment ranged from 24 hours to 4 days and dosages ranged from 7.5 mg to 60 mg daily. Overall bleeding rates were 2.5% in the ketorolac group compared with 2.1% in the control.[16] However, it should be noted that when combined with an epidural, ketorolac can put patients at risk for an epidural hematoma. The risk of NSAID administration in these cases has not been extensively studied, but there have been case reports; its mechanism of decreased

platelet aggregation gives plausibility to this theory.[17,18]

Local agents are also frequently used for pain control in body contouring procedures. A contin-uous epidural may be used before induction of anesthesia, which provides a combination of narcotic and local anesthesia components for the duration of the procedure. This practice is commonly used as part of the Enhanced Recovery After Surgery protocol currently implanted in colo-rectal surgery across the country. An article pub-lished in 2013 described a Cochrane review of 9 randomized controlled trials comparing IV patient-controlled analgesia (PCA) to continuous epidural analgesia. Patients with a continuous epidural had better pain control within the first 72 hours. Disadvantages are difficulty placing the epidural, failure of adequate pain control in 27% and 32% of lumbar and thoracic epidurals respectively.[19]

PROCEDURE-SPECIFIC RECOMMENDATIONS
Liposuction

Harvesting autologous fat for grafting using lipo-suction is currently the standard for reconstruction of soft tissue defects. It is also used as a body con-touring procedure to achieve decreased body mass in areas such as the thighs and abdomen. Tumescent anesthesia is commonly used with infusion of large volumes of solution containing a local anesthetic with epinephrine. It was popular-ized in 1994 by a dermatologist named Dr Jeffrey A. Klein, adopted from the older technique of massive infiltration analgesia with weak analgesic solutions from the 1910s.[20] The purpose of this technique is to allow liposuction to be performed under local anesthesia with virtually no blood loss. The package insert label on lidocaine with epinephrine states the maximum dose is 7 mg/kg for local infiltration. The liposuction guidelines of the American Society for Dermatologic Surgery cites the maximal safe dose for tumescent anes-thesia using lidocaine and epinephrine as 55 mg/kg. Tumescent solution contains at most 1g of lidocaine and 1 mg of epinephrine per liter of saline for a final lidocaine concentration of 0.9 g/L or 0.09%.[21] Because large volumes of this solution are removed almost immediately after infiltration and before absorption, the maximum dose can be much higher. The threshold for serum concen-tration of lidocaine is 6 µL/mL, after which patients begin to experience toxicity. In a later study by Klein and Jeske,[21] serum concentration of lido-caine was studied at intervals during liposuction procedures using large-volume (≥500 mL) tumes-cent infiltration. Postoperative patient monitoring included a physical examination and continuous heart rate, rhythm, pulse oximetry, and blood pressure measurements. After analyzing data comparing the total amount of lidocaine used and serum concentration, the investigators determined a reasonable maximum dose to be 45 mg/kg.

Tumescent anesthesia allows for postoperative pain control as well as improved ease of fat removal and has become the standard of care. Tumescent anesthesia with lidocaine provides peak plasma lidocaine concentrations at 12 to 14 hours after the start of infiltration and anesthesia for up to 18 hours. However, peak concentration depends on location as well. After injection into the thigh, maximum concentration occurred at 12 hours, whereas it occurred at up to 17 hours after injection in the abdominal wall. Complications are infrequent. In a questionnaire given to 66 surgeons who had performed liposuction with lidocaine on a total of 15,336 patients, there were no serious complications, such as death, embolism, hypovolemic shock, or thrombophlebitis. In another study of 688 patients, the rate of minor complications was 0.57%.[22]

A proposed disadvantage of lidocaine use in tumescent fluid is its inverse effect on cytotoxicity of adipose stem cells (ASCs). The average percentage of live in vitro ASCs in lidocaine-free solution vs tumescent solution with lidocaine was 86.7% and 68.0% respectively. This finding is a double-edged sword, as fat grafting is notorious for volume loss; therefore, this is an advantageous outcome. However, in liposuction for mass reduction this may be more favorable. This study also examined the difference between lidocaine and ropivacaine, which showed no difference in ASC survival. Lidocaine has a negative effect on ASC survival; absence improved stromal vascular fraction, which is especially important when used for fat grafting.[23]

Belt Lipectomy

Circumferential belt lipectomy is used for lower truncal remodeling. The procedure is a combination of traditional abdominoplasty and circumferential excision of skin and fat. Postoperative pain management is difficult because of the extensive surgical field and tension on the anterior and posterior suture lines, which may lead to wound dehiscence. Traditional oral analgesia in the form of opiates and NSAIDs may be used in addition to local anesthesia. One study analyzing the efficacy of the epidural in belt lipectomies found that in 62 patients undergoing these procedures, the average and maximum pain scores as well as

opioid usage were significantly lower in the experimental group. Before surgery, an epidural was placed in the lower thoracic region and infusion was initiated intraoperatively consisting of a combination of local and opiate analgesia. In postoperative days 0 and 1, the mean pain score was 1.53 and 1.84 on the visual analog scale versus 3.64 and 3.60 in the control group, respectively. The mean nonepidural opioid totals in morphine equivalents were 2.0 and 18.0 during postoperative days 0 and 1, respectively, in the cohort with an epidural versus 17.0 and 27.3 in the control group. The most significant drawbacks to an epidural are ease and reliability of placement. This drawback is especially true in patients undergoing belt lipectomies because they tend to have an unsuitable body habitus.[24]

Panniculectomy and Abdominoplasty

Like belt lipectomy, abdominoplasty alone is associated with serious discomfort. The ability to decrease pain is known to decrease hospital stay and allow for early mobilization, therefore, preventing thromboembolism. Regional infusion pumps with local anesthetic were introduced in the 1950s, but they were bulky and difficult to use. In 2005, these pain pumps became smaller, more precise, and disposable making them more popular and easy to use. In a randomized controlled trial, 20 female patients underwent abdominoplasty with rectus plication. Two groups were randomly divided, with the experimental group receiving a disposable incisional pain pump (Stryker Pain Pump 2, Kalamazoo, MI). This pump provided continuous delivery of 0.5% bupivacaine placed directly on top of the abdominal fascia. The pump can deliver infusion rates of 0.5 to 10.0 mL/h. Postoperatively, patients with the pain pump were able to ambulate 21.6 hours after surgery versus 40.8 hours in the control group. Patients consumed less postoperative narcotics in the experimental group as well.[25]

Despite promising results, pain pumps, such as the Stryker Pain Pump, On-Q (Irvine, CA), and Arrow Autofuser (Morrisville, NC), are still expensive and may be difficult to place. Catheters often move, as they are not secured; as mentioned earlier, the solution bathes the area of incision without promising the local anesthesia will be evenly dispersed. Closed suction drains often used in abdominoplasties may also affect this technique. An alternative to this approach is a transverse abdominus plane block performed intraoperatively. Another combination that has been reported is dilute local anesthesia used along the incision as well as high volumes injected into the fascia, thus, allowing the procedure to be performed under conscious sedation. Injections of 0.5% lidocaine with epinephrine has also been injected directly into the nerves as they perforate the rectus fascia. Patient satisfaction after this technique was high stating they would undergo cosmetic procedures with conscious sedation again when appropriate. It should be noted that the investigators dissuaded readers from using conscious sedation for patients with American Society of Anesthesiologists status greater than II.[26] A retrospective study of patients undergoing abdominoplasty with or without coprocedures, including liposuction, breast augmentation, mastopexy, capsulotomy, and varied facial procedures, examined the efficacy of local blocks as well. The investigator's technique was to perform intercostal blocks from T7 to T12 as well as blocks targeting the iliohypogastric and ilioinguinal nerves. A pararectus block was performed from the costal margin to the groin in the space between the internal oblique and transverse abdominis muscles. Procedure combinations were delineated by severity with the lowest being abdominoplasty alone increasing with the morbidity of coprocedures. Patients had lower pain scores and opiate use in the PACU across all severity classes.[27]

Breast Augmentation and Augmentation Mastopexy

As discussed earlier, breast augmentation is an opportunity to provide superior pain relief with local anesthetic to decrease opiate use. There have been promising results with the use of pain pumps for reconstructive procedures. A study of patients with and without pain pumps undergoing transverse rectus abdominis muscle flap reconstruction showed patients with local infiltration had lower PCA requirements and average days to discharge.[28] Although less than expected, a study from the University of Missouri showed marginally decreased pain scores in patients with an active pain pump. Twenty women were enrolled to receive a 4-day continuous infusion of bupivacaine with a pain pump in one breast pocket and a pain pump with saline in the other. Patients completed a questionnaire on postoperative days 1, 2, 3, 4, and 7. On all days, the mean pain scores were somewhat decreased on the experimental side in relation to the control. Despite the statistically insignificant results, patients reported they would use the pain pump again in future procedures.

REFERENCES

1. Sim R, Cheong DM, Wong KS, et al. Prospective randomized, double-blind, placebo-controlled study of pre- and postoperative administration of a COX-2-specific inhibitor as opioid-sparing analgesia in major colorectal surgery. Colorectal Dis 2007;9(1):52–60.

2. Karha J, Topol EJ. The sad story of Vioxx, and what we should learn from it. Cleve Clin J Med 2004;71(12):933–4.

3. Ross JS, Krumholz HM. Bringing Vioxx back to market. BMJ 2018;360:k242.

4. Sun T, Sacan O, White PF, et al. Perioperative versus postoperative celecoxib on patient outcomes after major plastic surgery procedures. Anesth Analg 2008;106(3):950–8.

5. Sardo P, Walker JH. Bariatric surgery: impact on medication management. Hosp Pharm 2008;43(2):113–20. Available at: http://ovidsp.ovid.com/ovidweb.cgi?T=JS&PAGE=reference&D=emed8&NEWS=N&AN=2009374535.

6. Murray M, Haiavy J. Preoperative intravenous acetaminophen improves recovery time after abdominoplasty. Am J Cosmet Surg 2015;32(3):144–8.

7. Moon YE, Lee YK, Lee J, et al. The effects of preoperative intravenous acetaminophen in patients undergoing abdominal hysterectomy. Arch Gynecol Obstet 2011;284(6):1455–60.

8. Fusco NM, Parbuoni K, Morgan JA. Drug utilization, dosing, and costs after implementation of intravenous acetaminophen guidelines for pediatric patients. J Pediatr Pharmacol Ther 2014;19(1):35–41.

9. Chaparro LE, Clarke H, Valdes PA, et al. Adding pregabalin to a multimodal analgesic regimen does not reduce pain scores following cosmetic surgery: a randomized trial. J Anesth 2012;26(6):829–35.

10. Zhang J, Ho KY, Wang Y. Efficacy of pregabalin in acute postoperative pain: a meta-analysis. Br J Anaesth 2011;106(4):454–62.

11. Peng PWH, Wijeysundera DN, Li CCF. Use of gabapentin for perioperative pain control - a meta-analysis. Pain Res Manag 2007;12(2):85–92.

12. Myles PS, Hendrata M, Bennett AM, et al. Postoperative nausea and vomiting. Propofol or thiopentone: does choice of induction agent affect outcome? Anaesth Intensive Care 1996;24(3):355–9.

13. Morales R, Mentz H, Newall G, et al. Use of abdominal field block injections with liposomal bupivacaine to control postoperative pain after abdominoplasty. Aesthet Surg J 2013;33(8):1148–53.

14. Vyas KS, Rajendran S, Morrison SD, et al. Systematic review of liposomal bupivacaine (Exparel) for postoperative analgesia. Plast Reconstr Surg 2016;138(4):748e–56e.

15. Maund E, McDaid C, Rice S, et al. Paracetamol and selective and non-selective non-steroidal anti-inflammatory drugs for the reduction in morphine-related side-effects after major surgery: a systematic review. Br J Anaesth 2011;106(3):292–7.

16. Gobble RM, Hoang HLT, Kachniarz B, et al. Ketoro-lac does not increase perioperative bleeding: a meta-analysis of randomized controlled trials. Plast Reconstr Surg 2014;133(3):741–55.

17. Jeon DG, Song JG, Kim S-K, et al. Epidural hema-toma after thoracic epidural analgesia in a patient treated with ketorolac, mefenamic acid, and nafta-zone: a case report. Korean J Anesthesiol 2014; 66(3):240.

18. Chang Chien GC, McCormick Z, Araujo M, et al. The potential contributing effect of ketorolac and fluoxe-tine to a spinal epidural hematoma following a cervi-cal interlaminar epidural steroid injection: a case report and narrative review. Pain Physician 2014; 17(3):E385–95.

19. Garimella V, Cellini CM. Postoperative pain control. Clin Colon Rectal Surg 2013;26(3):191–6.

20. Welch JD. History of tumescent anesthesia, part i: from American Surgical Textbooks of the 1920s and 1930s. Aesthet Surg J 1998;18(5):353–7.

21. Klein JA, Jeske DR. Estimated maximal safe dos-ages of tumescent lidocaine. Anesth Analg 2016; 122(5):1350–9.

22. Kompardt J, Schug S. Local anesthetics. In: Aron-son J, editor. Side effects of drugs annual. 34th edi-tion. Elsevier 2012:209–22.

23. Goldman JJ, Wang WZ, Fang X-H, et al. Tumescent liposuction without lidocaine. Plast Reconstr Surg Glob Open 2016;4(8):e829.

24. Michaud A-P, Rosenquist RW, Cram AE, et al. An evaluation of epidural analgesia following circumfer-ential belt lipectomy. Plast Reconstr Surg 2007; 120(2):538–44.

25. Mentz HA, Ruiz-Razura A, Newall G, et al. Use of a regional infusion pump to control postoperative pain after an abdominoplasty. Aesthetic Plast Surg 2005;29(5):415–21.

26. Kryger ZB, Fine NA, Mustoe TA. The outcome of ab-dominoplasty performed under conscious sedation: six-year experience in 153 consecutive cases. Plast Reconstr Surg 2004;113(6):1807–17.

27. Feng LJ. Painless abdominoplasty: the efficacy of combined intercostal and pararectus blocks in reducing postoperative pain and recovery time. Plast Reconstr Surg 2010;126(5):1723–32.

28. Losken A, Parris JJ, Douglas TD, et al. Use of the infusion pain pump following transverse rectus ab-dominis muscle flap breast reconstruction. Ann Plast Surg 2005;54(5):479–82.

Abdominal Contouring and Combining Procedures

Tali Friedman, MD, MHA[a],*, Itay Wiser, MD, PhD[b,c]

KEYWORDS

- Abdominal contouring • Combined procedures • Surgical technique • Patient safety

KEY POINTS

- The initial evaluation of patients with massive weight loss (MWL) must include a thorough physical, medical, and mental assessment.
- In order to maximize the safety of the procedure, patients with MWL should be offered a staged surgical plan.
- An accurate assessment of the patients' preferences and concerns, followed by realistic expectations for the procedure, are key components to achieving optimal patient satisfaction.
- Using conservative liposuction in abdominoplasty is safe and highly recommended for aesthetic reasons; it contributes to improved tissue redraping, minimizing epigastric and upper rolls volume and allows less midline undermining.
- Potential dead-space suture closure allows for better healing and minimal use of drains.

 Video content accompanies this article at http://www.plasticsurgery.theclinics.com/.

INTRODUCTION

Obesity affects the abdominal area causing irreversible skeletal and soft tissue deformities that can currently only be modified surgically.[1]

The extent and type of abdominoplasty, which is designed for a specific patient, depends on certain anatomic components of the abdomen, including the amount of skin and quality, fat distribution, diastasis recti width, location, and muscle tone. Other factors are body proportions, amount of upper transverse redundancy in relation to interflank width, height of rolls deformity and adhesion lines, as well as the amount of skin deformity at adjacent areas, such as the lateral thighs, flanks, and buttocks. Other important parameters are the existence of old abdominal scars; abdominal hernias; amount of intra-abdominal fat; patients' body mass index (BMI); patients' health; smoking

status; individual risk of poor scarring; and acceptance of scars, length, and location.

The authors would like to emphasize 5 key points to a comprehensive surgical approach of the abdomen in patients with MWL[1]: comprehensive preoperative patient evaluation[2]; matching the abdominoplasty technique to the specific patient[3]; abdominal contouring and combined procedures[4]; technical pearls in MWL abdominoplasty[5]; patient safety and risk assessment.

PREOPERATIVE PATIENT EVALUATION
Patient Selection

Abdominoplasty is a very gratifying procedure, which may come with specific side effects and complications (**Box 1**). In order to lower the complication rate, a thorough patient evaluation should be done at the first patient consultation,

The authors have nothing to disclose.

[a] The Body Contouring Center, 47 Brodezky Street, Tel- Aviv, Israel; [b] Department of Epidemiology and Preventive Medicine, Sackler Faculty of Medicine, Tel-Aviv University, Tel-Aviv, Israel; [c] Department of Plastic Surgery, Lenox Hill Hospital, New York, NY, USA
* Corresponding author.
E-mail address: Drtali@talifriedman.com

Clin Plastic Surg 46 (2019) 41–48
https://doi.org/10.1016/j.cps.2018.08.006

Box 1
**Comprehensive preoperative patients'
evaluation**

- Thorough patient evaluations are conducted
  to rule out risk factors for complications.
- Active smoking is detrimental to wound healing and should be discontinued 1 month
  before surgery.
- Weight stability is evaluated and discussed.
- Safety guidelines are personalized.
- Postoperative hematocrit level is the most
  important factor for recovery.

with emphasis on the anatomic structure of the
abdomen as well as medical status, smoking history, and personal expectations. Risk factors for
wound healing complications are specifically evaluated. They include smoking, diabetes, hypertension,
asthma, and hypothyroidism. These risk factors
should be followed and controlled before surgery.

Patients with MWL often take antidepressant
medications; but very rarely, they are not suitable
for a skin reduction procedure. The authors ask for
psychiatric clearance only to those who are being
actively treated by a psychiatrist or psychologist.

The authors discuss exercise and diet routines
with all their new patients while highlighting health-
ier behavior. Weight stability is discussed as well,
and the authors recommend at least 3 months of
stability before any skin reduction procedure.
There is no clear definition regarding the stability
of weight. In the authors' practice, they define stability as a 1-kg change in a month.

In the authors' practice, they recommend
combining as many procedures as possible in a single stage, within safety guidelines. These safety
guidelines includes preoperative hematocrit level,
amount of potential bleeding (extensiveness of liposuction, pannus volume, number of surgical sites,
and so forth), physical fitness, age (70 years or older
will have only one area operated on at a time), current
BMI (BMI 32–35, only one area operated), support
group, mental status, normal laboratory tests, and
so forth. Postoperative hematocrit level is the single
most important factor influencing recovery and early
ambulation. Therefore, it is crucial to test the hematocrit early in the patients' evaluation and consider
hematocrit elevation by IV or oral iron supplements
according to the extent of the surgical plan.

Physical Examination and Abdominal Assessment

Body morphometry and proportions should be evaluated during the initial patient consultation (**Box 2**).

Three-dimensional skeletal proportions and
asymmetries influence the abdominal shape. Skeletal deformities of the ribs, pelvic bones, and
midline are very common among patients with
MWL[1]; these include anterior pelvis tilt, prominent
rib cage and prominent xyphoid, pelvic asymmetries, and umbilical malposition.

Recognizing the skeletal body habitus is crucial
in order to predict whether the waistline will be
emphasized or not after surgery, and this should
be made clear to patients before surgery.

Chronic and repetitive expansions of the intra-
abdominal contents lead to irrepressible
spreading and distraction of the abdominal wall
lamellas. All these layers of tissues should be
evaluated at the initial patient consultation. The
deepest abdominal wall lamella includes the
muscular-fascial layer. Muscle tone should be
evaluated as well as width and height of diastasis
recti. Intra-abdominal fat should be differentiated
from muscle diastasis based on a physical examination. The binder test assists in differentiating
between high abdominal pressures due to intra-
abdominal fat or due to muscle diastasis. It includes wearing the binder for a month preoperatively. Patients with severe diastasis will be able
to decrease abdominal prominence by using the
tight binder, as opposed to high intra-abdominal
obese patients who will not improve. Umbilical
and postoperative ventral hernias are very common in MWL and should be recognized
preoperatively.

The second abdominal wall lamella includes the
fat layers and the superficial fascia. The fat layers'
depth should be evaluated, specifically the deep
fat layer, and the extent of liposuction estimated,
specifically at the epigastric and on the upper rib
cage areas, as these areas tend to be neglected
often and tend to become prominent postoperatively. The extent of epigastric liposuction should
be limited and be done for the most part deep
and conservatively, specifically in smokers and
high BMI patients, because aggressive epigastric
liposuction is a known risk factor for flap ischemia
and necrosis.[2]

The superficial, third lamella of the abdominal
wall consists of the skin. This layer significantly influences the long-term abdominal aesthetic result
and should be evaluated in a 3-dimensional
manner.

The amount of epigastric skin and umbilical
height are important factors that influence the possibility of a vertical lower abdominal scar, and this
should be emphasized on the consent form. Dou-
ble- or 3-roll deformities and adhesion lines are
important in discussing the fleur-de-lis (FDL) technique versus the standard abdominoplasty. When

---

Box 2
Physical examination and abdominal assessment

- Three-dimensional skeletal evaluation
- Body habitus and proportions
- Amount of intra-abdominal fat
- Evaluation of fascia-muscular lamella
- Three-dimensional evaluation of skin redundancy and elasticity
- Abdominal wall scars: quality, location, tethered
- Evaluation of mons deformity

---

there is good skin elasticity, liposuction of the upper third roll and unfurling the deep fibrotic adhesions is enough for roll elimination in most cases. However, with poor skin elasticity, only direct skin removal will eliminate that upper roll. In this stage, the advantages of the FDL technique are emphasized to patients. When poor skin elasticity is recognized, the probability of a second complementary procedure should be emphasized as well in the initial consult.

The severity of mons deformity should be evaluated in terms of vertical ptosis, transverse width, and fat deposition.[3]

High intra-abdominal fat is a risk factor for recurrence epigastric prominence, and this should be thoroughly explained to patients before surgery. It should be recommended to patients with high intra-abdominal fat to lose more weight before surgery, no matter what their BMI actually may be. Practically, the pannus dimensions has much less impact on the aesthetic result, as opposed to the intra-abdominal fat and epigastric skin quality and quantity. Epigastric striae is a sign of poor skin elasticity and is a risk factor for secondary skin redundancy.[4]

Abdominal hernias should be ruled out by a physical examination and radiographic imaging if needed. However, postoperative hernias are very common in patients with postbariatric MWL and should be watched during surgery regardless.

MATCHING THE ABDOMINOPLASTY TECHNIQUE TO PATIENTS

The first decision when planning abdominal contouring surgery is to decide which abdominal contouring technique fits the patients' anatomic deformity and aesthetic expectations, with minimal risks. The alternative techniques that are relevant to the abdomen of patients with MWL are

panniculectomy (removal of skin below the umbilicus) and standard abdominoplasty, reverse abdominoplasty, and FDL-abdominoplasty. The type of procedure chosen is based on a combination of factors, leading up to a definite decision, which is made together with patients.

Panniculectomy is often considered as a functional surgery, usually offered to patients with a high BMI who have high intra-abdominal fat with and reasonable expectations. It is a very gratifying procedure in this group of patients. However, these patients are always offered other alternatives as well, considering their ability to further lose weight.

Interestingly, there are some aesthetic indications to the classic panniculectomy, even in patients with very high expectations who have the combination of high umbilicus and fear of umbilical scar, or as a revision surgery in patients who already have had abdominoplasty years ago and wish to lower or improve their old abdominal scar. This procedure can also be combined with a lower body lift (LBL) (**Fig. 1**).

The FDL abdominoplasty is a very useful technique in controlling significant transverse skin redundancy in the epigastric area when patients desire to be as tight as possible, understanding the trade-off of a vertical midline scar.

However, many variables influence the final decision and, therefore, are discussed with patients before the final decision is made. The patients' preferred aesthetic and functional needs are analyzed together with the objective parameters of skin quality, roll location, and severity of skin redundancy in proportion to body morphometry.[5]

FDL abdominoplasty is a very safe and gratifying technique with very high patient satisfaction; its only disadvantage is the midline scar, though keeping the midline perforators will lower the risk of tissue ischemia as already described.[6]

Decision-making is based on the amount of transverse skin redundancy, many times presented as medial upper roll, skin quality, and aesthetic priorities of the authors' patients. The main trade-off is the midline scar; many times patients prefer a lower aesthetic result of this scar. Therefore, the best candidates for the FDL-abdominoplasty are patients with significant upper abdominal scars and patients with high medial roll and significant upper transverse redundancy with poor elasticity (striae) (**Fig. 2**).

However, a pleasant aesthetic result is often reached in patients with upper transverse redundancy by standard abdominoplasty only, by wider undermining and skin redraping, unfurling the upper roll, and conservative liposuction. This technique works better with good skin elasticity and

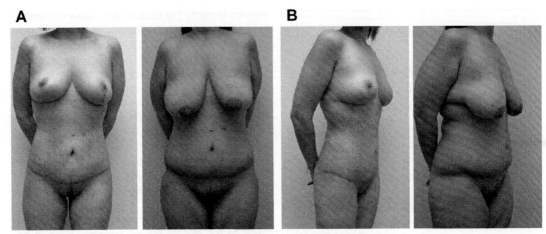

Fig. 1. A 23 year old who lost 80 kg and had 2-stage TBL: upper body lift (*A*) and LBL (*B*), including vertical thigh-plasty. The LBL included only panniculectomy, as she disliked the umbilical scar.

specifically in the gynoid morphometry, with a wide interpelvic width as opposed to a thin waist.

About 5% of the abdominoplasty patients in the authors' clinic will have the FDL abdominoplasty, even after the alternative has been discussed with them preoperatively. Being offered the transverse tightening will stay in their mind, and they will be more understanding after the surgery when they recognize some secondary redundancy when edema resolves.

Reverse abdominoplasty is a technique with limited yield in the long run and, therefore, is reserved mainly for patients who already have inframammary scars. The authors offer this procedure as a secondary tightening procedure to control upper lateral rolls.

Single Versus Multiple Areas Procedures

Objectively, many body areas represent redundant skin after weight loss; however, not all the patients will proceed to a total makeover. The most common reason for choosing only one area is financial.[7–10]

In most patients who proceed on to a total body lift, the common practice is a staged fashion, including as many anatomic areas as possible at a time. This approach has many advantages, as it contributes to a total change in 2 to 3 stages, most often in less than a year, with aesthetic, financial, and even medical advantages.[11]

Poor skin elasticity, which is the common trait in patients with MWL, is the leading cause for

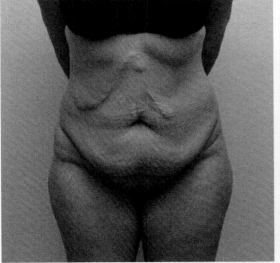
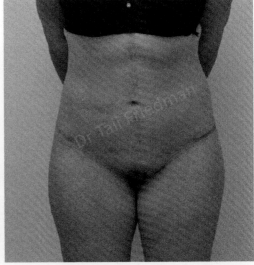

Fig. 2. A 42 year old who lost 40 kg (BMI 25) and was a smoker. She had old upper abdominal scars. She had an FDL-LBL.

A **B**

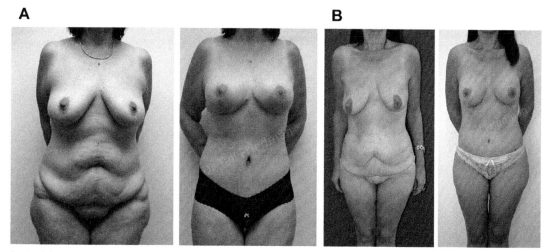

Fig. 3. (*A*) A 45 year old who lost 100 kg and had a mastopexy and LBL as a single procedure. (*B*) A 40 year old who lost 75 kg. She had 2-stage TBL: LBL and mastopexy-augmentation and brachioplasty and vertical thigh-plasty.

patients' disappointment in the long run. Therefore, the opportunity to revise a scar to improve tightness during another procedure is gratifying for patients. Therefore, the authors highly recommend waiting at least 6 months between the first and the last elective surgeries to evaluate if significant skin redundancy has developed.

There are recent data showing that body-contouring surgeries contribute to better weight control after MWL.[12–14] The impact of these surgeries becomes even more important as the authors' understand the high rate of bariatric surgery's long-term failure.[15,16] Additionally, the authors have currently demonstrated that the extensiveness of the anatomic areas operated is correlated with the patients' ability to maintain their weight in the long run and even assists them in losing more weight if more than 3 anatomic areas have been operated on.[12]

In the multiple-procedures group in the authors' cohort, the most common combination is abdominoplasty or LBL with a breast aesthetic surgery (62% of the patients), the most common was mastopexy (**Fig. 3**). The prevalence of the upper body lift (UBL) is 20% among the first-stage procedures (**Fig. 4**, Video 1).

TECHNICAL PEARLS IN ABDOMINOPLASTY

Liposuction is a very important tool when combined with abdominoplasty. It decreases fat collection in tissue folds; but more importantly, it assists in the redraping of the whole abdominal skin, even with limited midline undermining.

The tissue-closing technique is based on the understanding that the obliteration of dead space is

mandatory for a better healing process. In the past, few drains were left in each LBL procedure. In patients who had had further revision abdominoplasty, one can notice often a deep seroma capsule even many years after. Progressive tissue sutures decrease the rate of early and late healing complications, such as expanding hematomas, chronic seroma pockets, and long-standing drains. Another important advantage of the progressive sutures is the reduction of ischemia and necrosis, as tension is divided along the flap. However, for safety measures, a drain is left in for the first few days.

The flap measurement and trimming is completed before the progressive tension sutures are put in place. The authors use 0 polyglactin (Vicryl, Ethicon Inc, Somerville, NJ) stiches and include the superficial fascia with the stich but not the dermis. Care must be taken in patients with very thin subcutaneous tissue, specifically with the midline stiches, to prevent ischemia due to close midline stiches.

Seventy percent of the abdominal contouring procedures in the authors' cohort are part of LBL. Most of them include the conventional buttock transverse incisions (95%). About 2% of the LBL will have versatile elliptical excisions at the back due to a combination of transverse and vertical redundancy of fibrotic tissues (**Fig. 5**).

PERIOPERATIVE ABDOMINOPLASTY SAFETY MEASURES

The authors operate in a medical center where patients are discharged after 23 hours. The ability to operate on multiple areas at a time and send

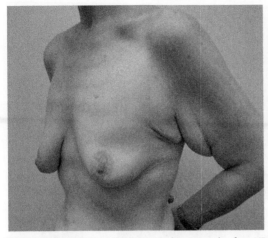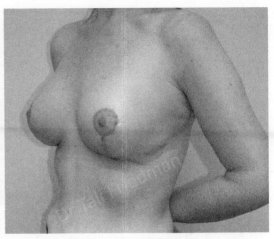

Fig. 4. A 40 year old who lost 110 kg; 1 week after UBL as the first stage of TBL reconstruction.

patients home after 23 hours is based on their ability to lower side effects and complication rates. The most important parameter that correlates with early ambulation is postoperative hematocrit. Its value is influenced from the preoperative hematocrit level and amount of bleeding during and after surgery. Therefore, the authors put some effort into elevating hematocrit before surgery with iron supplements if needed and to lower the intraoperative and postoperative bleeding as much as possible. During the surgery, attention is given to decrease bleeding using hemostatic solutions, liposuction instead of direct incision if possible, elimination of dead spaces, and meticulous hemostasis of surgical planes. Cooperation with the anesthesiologist is mandatory for blood pressure control throughout the surgery and after. Many of the expanding hematomas start when patients experience elevated blood pressure due to pain or anxiety very early after surgery; therefore, meticulous control of blood pressure starts before the extubation.

Venous thromboembolic event prevention is done by a combination of sequential compression devices starting before induction, early ambulation, and subcutaneous Enoxaparin 40 to 60 mg starting the morning after surgery, for at least 2 weeks after every abdominoplasty. Because 50% of the first deep venous thrombosis events occur in patients with no history of thrombophilia, every patient having abdominoplasty is considered a moderate-risk patient and should be treated for at least 2 weeks postoperatively.[17,18]

The length of surgery is another factor, which correlates with postoperative complications. The authors try to limit the combined surgery length to 5 hours at the most.

Hypothermia prevention is another important factor meticulously controlled in combined surgeries. The authors warm their patients in the

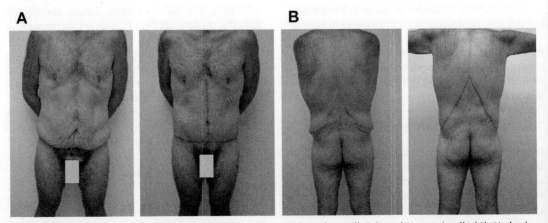

Fig. 5. A 38 year old who lost 110 kg. He asked for one procedure that will tighten him maximally (*A*). He had an FDL-LBL, with posterior oblique incisions for maximal, multi-vector lift (*B*).

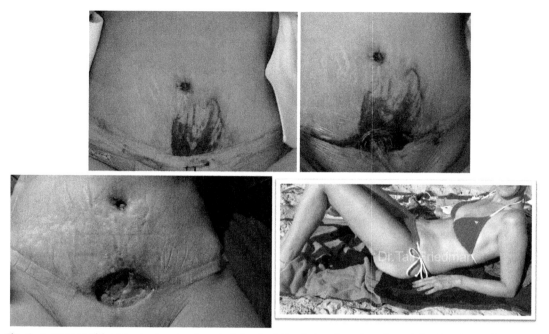

Fig. 6. A 32-year-old patient who developed abdominal flap ischemia a day after abdominoplasty. The patient was treated with HBOT and negative pressure dressing for several weeks. All demarcated areas survived, and the surgical wound was closed in the office a month after surgery.

presurgery holding area and use warm fluids, warming blankets, and warming sheets throughout surgery.

Hyperbaric oxygen therapy (HBOT): In the last 5 years, the use of preoperative and postoperative HBOT has become very common for patients in the authors' clinic, for variable indications. Preconditioning by preoperative HBOT was shown to decrease the ischemic complications of standard abdominoplasty.[19] Therefore, the authors send active smokers for 1 to 2 treatments before the surgery, after lowering the smoking amount significantly. If needed, the authors use a few treatments immediately after. Other high-risk patients can reap the benefits from HBOT before surgery, such as patients who need significant epigastric liposuction or very wide undermining. The preconditioning concept was developed secondary to the authors' experience with HBOT treating ischemic flap complications (**Fig. 6**).

Another indication for HBOT is vertical thighplasty. The groin area tends to heal slower than other areas because of maceration and infection. Better tissue oxygenation and early edema reduction improves healing in these patients. Therefore, these patients are routinely offered 3 postoperative HBOTs.

Optimal scar treatment: About 90% of the authors' patients choose at least one scar treatment modality. The most common treatment is silicon

sheets. The second most common treatment is lasers. Thirty percent of the patients will use silicone sheets and lasers. The scar revision rate has dropped to less than 1% since lasers have become part of the regular scar management protocol.

SUMMARY

Being able to combine different surgical sites together with abdominoplasty is a mandatory approach for patients with MWL. It is highly recommended to start with the abdomen as the first stage, combined with other surgical sites, in order to limit the total body reconstruction to 2 surgical stages. The surgical plan is influenced by personal, clinical, medical, and financial parameters and is always individualized.

SUPPLEMENTARY DATA

Supplementary data related to this article can be found online at https://doi.org/10.1016/j.cps.2018.08.006.

REFERENCES

1. Song AY, Jean RD, Hurwitz DJ, et al. A classification of contour deformities after bariatric weight loss: the Pittsburgh Rating Scale. Plast Reconstr Surg 2005;116(5):1535–44 [discussion: 45–6].

2. Michaels Jt, Coon D, Rubin JP. Complications in postbariatric body contouring: strategies for assessment and prevention. Plast Reconstr Surg 2011; 127(3):1352–7.

3. Michaels JT, Friedman T, Coon D, et al. Mons rejuvenation in the massive weight loss patient using superficial fascial system suspension. Plast Reconstr Surg 2010;126(1):45e–6e.

4. Almutairi K, Gusenoff JA, Rubin JP. Body contouring. Plast Reconstr Surg 2016;137(3):586e–602e.

5. Bossert RP, Rubin JP. Evaluation of the weight loss patient presenting for plastic surgery consultation. Plast Reconstr Surg 2012;130(6):1361–9.

6. Friedman T, O'Brien Coon D, Michaels J, et al. Fleur-de-Lis abdominoplasty: a safe alternative to traditional abdominoplasty for the massive weight loss patient. Plast Reconstr Surg 2010;125(5):1525–35.

7. Kitzinger HB, Abayev S, Pittermann A, et al. The prevalence of body contouring surgery after gastric bypass surgery. Obes Surg 2012;22(1):8–12.

8. Mitchell JE, Crosby RD, Ertelt TW, et al. The desire for body contouring surgery after bariatric surgery. Obes Surg 2008;18(10):1308–12.

9. Sioka E, Tzovaras G, Katsogridaki G, et al. Desire for body contouring surgery after laparoscopic sleeve gastrectomy. Aesthetic Plast Surg 2015;39(6): 978–84.

10. Steffen KJ, Sarwer DB, Thompson JK, et al. Predictors of satisfaction with excess skin and desire for body contouring after bariatric surgery. Surg Obes Relat Dis 2012;8(1):92–7.

11. Coon D, Michaels Jt, Gusenoff JA, et al. Multiple procedures and staging in the massive weight loss population. Plast Reconstr Surg 2010;125(2):691–8.

12. Wiser I, Heller L, Spector C, et al. Body contouring procedures in three or more anatomical areas are associated with long-term body mass index decrease in massive weight loss patients: a retrospective cohort study. J Plast Reconstr Aesthet Surg 2017;70(9):1181–5.

13. Wiser I, Avinoah E, Ziv O, et al. Body contouring surgery decreases long-term weight regain following laparoscopic adjustable gastric banding: a matched retrospective cohort study. J Plast Reconstr Aesthet Surg 2016;69(11):1490–6.

14. Balague N, Combescure C, Huber O, et al. Plastic surgery improves long-term weight control after bariatric surgery. Plast Reconstr Surg 2013;132(4): 826–33.

15. Boza C, Gamboa C, Awruch D, et al. Laparoscopic Roux-en-Y gastric bypass versus laparoscopic adjustable gastric banding: five years of follow-up. Surg Obes Relat Dis 2010;6(5):470–5.

16. Weichman K, Ren C, Kurian M, et al. The effectiveness of adjustable gastric banding: a retrospective 6-year U.S. follow-up study. Surg Endosc 2011; 25(2):397–403.

17. Clavijo-Alvarez JA, Pannucci CJ, Oppenheimer AJ, et al. Prevention of venous thromboembolism in body contouring surgery: a national survey of 596 ASPS surgeons. Ann Plast Surg 2011;66(3): 228–32.

18. Friedman T, O'Brien Coon D, Michaels VJ, et al. Hereditary coagulopathies: practical diagnosis and management for the plastic surgeon. Plast Reconstr Surg 2010;125(5):1544–52.

19. Friedman T. Preconditioning with hyperbaric oxygenation reduces post abdominoplasty complications in high risk smoking population. The 3rd international conference on hyperbaric oxygen therapy and the brain, Eilat, Israel, May 18–19, 2017.

Fleur-de-lis Abdominoplasty and Neo-umbilicus

Flávio Henrique Mendes, MD, PhD*,
Alfredo Donnabella, MD, Alan Roberto Fagotti Moreira, MD

KEYWORDS

- Massive weight loss • Body contouring • Neo-umbilicoplasty • Post-bariatric
- Vertical abdominoplasty

KEY POINTS

- Post–bariatric surgery body contouring implies complete anatomic and functional readjustment of the entire superficial fascial system. Correction vectors should be considered both vertically and horizontally.
- It is reasonable that many of these patients demand not only lifting but also some extent of central body tightening, with vertical resections.
- Traditional outer scar umbilical techniques are associated with a wide source of complications, with bad scaring and shape distortions that represent important aesthetic drawbacks.
- Best umbilical reconstruction should consider anatomic landmarks, including base, grooving, and ring, all of them achieved by the inner scar umbilicoplasty.
- Especially for patients with massive weight loss, the new inner scar umbilicoplasty provides a unique and natural navel aspect, enhancing overall results for vertical approach abdominoplasties.

INTRODUCTION

Body contouring surgery has experienced a true resurgence with the popularization of the surgical treatment of morbid obesity. In the last 2 decades we have seen a new and growing population of patients with massive weight loss (MWL) showing extremely challenging deformities, demanding new approaches and techniques in search of better results. Unlike conventional patients, the particular physiopathology involved with these deformities requires careful observation by the specialist, while considering the specific anatomic changes and tissue biodynamics for improved diagnosis and surgical planning.

Furthermore, metabolic status of patients who lose weight must be considered in the face of the restrictive and/or dis-absorptive effects of bariatric procedures. Although the general condition and clinical comorbidities of obese patients show significant improvement after weight loss, different patterns of nutritional deficits may be found in the preoperative approach for body contouring.[1] Special clinical and laboratorial assessment in order to identify and correct those conditions are fundamental to optimize homeostasis and surgical wound healing on these patients.[2] Similarly, the psychological status of post–bariatric surgery patients deserves special attention because specific disorders are often associated and can negatively impact postoperative recovery. A multidisciplinary team approach is the gold standard in treating these patients from the beginning of their struggle

The authors have nothing to disclose.
Plastic Surgery Division, Botucatu Medical School, Paulista State University, Rua Tomaz Antonio Gonzaga, 160 Lins, São Paulo 16400-465, Brazil
* Corresponding author. Rua Tomaz Antonio Gonzaga, 160 Lins, São Paulo 16400-465, Brazil.
E-mail address: mendesmd@fhmendes.com.br

Clin Plastic Surg 46 (2019) 49–60
https://doi.org/10.1016/j.cps.2018.08.007

against obesity throughout weight stabilization and recovery of a better body shape.[3]

In order to achieve better results in post–bariatric surgery body contouring, it may be necessary to address both vertical and horizontal tissue excess, promoting not only a body lifting but also a tightening effect, which includes longitudinal resections over the trunk and limbs.[4] Specifically on the central/lower body, those resections usually end up with anterior vertical scars seen on the fleur-de-lis technique. Although achieving nice contouring results, poor visible scaring, including umbilical complications, have restricted the indications for the anterior vertical approach.[5] The purpose of this article is to present the authors' experience with the inner scar umbilical reconstruction, enhancing the overall results in vertical abdominoplasties.

PHYSIOPATHOLOGY OF THE MASSIVE WEIGHT LOSS DEFORMITIES

On a tomographic detailed research of the entire continuity of subcutaneous cellular tissue, Markman and Barton[6] stated the superficial fascia is a constant structure, dividing superficial and deep fat compartments throughout nearly all of the trunk and limbs. Avelar[7] observed fascial variations affecting layers and thickness in different areas of the body depending on regional amounts of fat. In 1991, Lockwood[8] published new concepts that provided a better and more complete understanding of the entire 3-dimensional structure of connective tissue within subcutaneous fat, defining and popularizing the so-called superficial fascial system (SFS), which is specifically responsible for supporting the skin tegument (**Fig. 1**A). Large accumulations in the adipocytes of obese patients create a generalized mechanical stretching effect in the SFS through volumetric increase of the whole subcutaneous space (**Fig. 1**B). Meanwhile, weight loss causes a massive adipocyte reduction reflecting volumetric deflation of the subcutaneous tissue without the retraction of collagen fibers, which remain elongated and weak (**Fig. 1**C). Ultimately, SFS disability leads to significant looseness of the cutaneous covering as a whole.

Following MWL, patients experience a generalized laxity with great mobility of covering tissue, which directly impacts body contour through the excess and selective descent of surrounding segments. The zones of adherence (**Fig. 2**) are extremely important in the final composition of human silhouette, because they promote a "selective limitation" in the mobility of skin coverage around the body.[9] The location and intensity of these subcutaneous adherences remain relatively constant in different individuals of both sexes, so that gravitational effect on different amounts of deflated tissue will determine individual contouring characteristics. In other words, the translational effect of mobile tissue in contrast to areas with greater deep fixation designs the contouring profile of post–bariatric surgery patients.[5] This idea is the fundamental anatomic rule that defines body contour deformities in the MWL population, determining a completely different approach, targeting the new biodynamics of the involved tissues.

CENTRAL AND LOWER BODY READJUSTMENT VECTORS

Keeping those physiopathology aspects in mind, body segments should be analyzed as cylinders for better understanding of excess tissue behavior. Although we see specific areas showing evident ptosis, due to gravitational restriction by the zones of adherence, lifting vectors may not be enough to correct the problem, which might need longitudinal resections with vertical (fleur-de-lis) or lateral approaches, considering the generalized and circumferential pattern of body deformities (**Fig. 3**).

Post–bariatric surgery body readjustment implies complete anatomic and functional readjustment of the entire superficial fascial system. Correction vectors should be considered both vertically and horizontally, understanding that horizontal resections generally promote a lift of tissues, whereas vertical ones promote a tighter coverage along the longitudinal axis. The combination of these two approaches provides the concept of body readjustment: lifting and tightening.[5] Although Rahban and Gross[10] suggested longitudinal tightening through bilateral resections placed at both axillary lines, the anterior midline approach known as *fleur-de-lis abdominoplasty* is much more popular, with or without circumferential belt lipectomies.

In this way, readjustment of the central/lower body means lifting the infero-anterior, lateral, and/or posterior segments but may also need a vertical tightening through longitudinal resections, generally placed along the anterior median line (**Fig. 4**). Physical examination with vigorous palpation is the gold standard tool to generally identify and quantify excess tissue, defining resection plans and correction vectors with complete understanding and agreement of patients.

DIAGNOSIS AND PLANNING

Physical examination of the lower body should begin with static inspection of standing patients, with the examiner seated on a swiveling stool

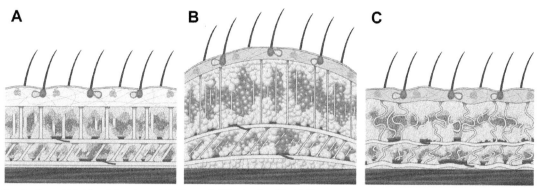

Fig. 1. Superficial fascial system. (*A*) Normal, (*B*) obesity, (*C*) MWL.

that permits free movement around patients. Wall mirrors should be available in the examination room because they allow the examiner to show and educate the patients about their whole extent of tissue laxity (mobility) as well as the recommended vectors for best contouring readjustment. Orthostatic folds and sulci should be identified around the circumference of the body, considering the physiopathology of MWL contour deformities. Vigorous palpation of the involved tissues helps to simulate the effects to be obtained with resection and potential correction vectors. Previous identification of scars and hernias in the abdominal wall is also essential in the planning and safety of the proposed treatment. Plication of the anterior aponeurosis should be performed as it goes in conventional surgery, usually necessary considering prior distension by intra-abdominal fat during obesity or even past pregnancies. Cases of small and uncomplicated hernias, with a ring of up to approximately 10 cm in diameter, may be simply corrected by the medial aponeurosis plication;

but in most difficult cases the use of alloplastic material is recommended (synthetic mesh). Usually, a regularly trained plastic surgeon is fully capable of conducting most of those treatments in the same approach, whereas more complex cases should be executed in cooperation with other specialists in abdominal wall reconstruction.

It is reasonable that post–bariatric surgery patients may demand not only lifting but also some extent of central body tightening, with vertical resections. Modolin and colleagues[11] published a wide systematization of possible approaches to abdominoplasty after MWL, including anterior transverse (conventional), anterior combined (fleur-de-lis), circumferential (belt), and circumferential combined (fleur-de-lis + belt).

Anterior Transverse Approach

The anterior transverse abdominoplasty, routinely used for conventional patients, is seldom recommended for the post–bariatric surgery population

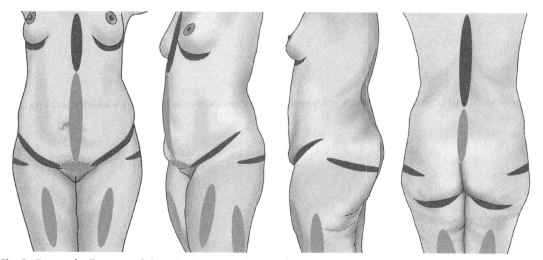

Fig. 2. Zones of adherence of the subcutaneous tissue. *Red*, strong; *green*, mild.

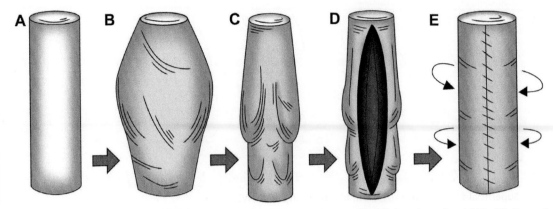

Fig. 3. Deflation and orthostatic biodynamic. The role of tissue longitudinal tightening after MWL. (*A*) Normal, (*B*) obese, (*C*) deflation, (*D, E*) longitudinal resection.

(**Fig. 5**A). Although it might be efficient to treat regular deformities resulting from multiple pregnancies, which are mainly restricted to the anterior aspect of the lower trunk, this technique tends to be insufficient for treating general MWL circumferential laxity. In most cases, the anterior transverse approach alone does not correct horizontal excess tissue in the upper abdomen as well as lateral and posterior ptosis (thighs, flanks, and buttocks), leading to residual laxity that is extremely inconvenient when body contouring is evaluated as a whole.

Circumferential Approach

The objective of this technique is to expand the anterior transverse resection of the lower abdomen to the flanks and lower dorsum, removing an actual belt of excess tissue to lift the anterior and lateral aspect of the thighs as well as the gluteal region (**Fig. 5**B). This procedure is especially indicated for patients with the peripheral pattern of fat deposits and offers excellent results by treating significant ptosis of the lateral and posterior structures of the lower body. In cases whereby fat deposits mainly occur above the waistline (central obesity), just like for the anterior transverse approach, it should be emphasized that the circumferential technique alone may not correct the horizontal excess in the upper abdomen and may result in greater or lesser levels of remaining anterior laxity.

Combined Anterior Approach

Also known as *anchor line* or *fleur-de-lis* abdominoplasty, this technique combines longitudinal resection with the anterior transverse approach specifically to address the horizontal excess abdominal tissue, which is normally present in

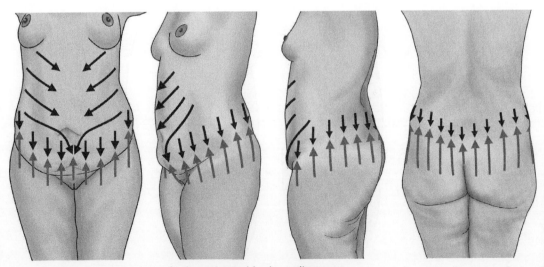

Fig. 4. Possible correction vectors for lower/central body readjustment.

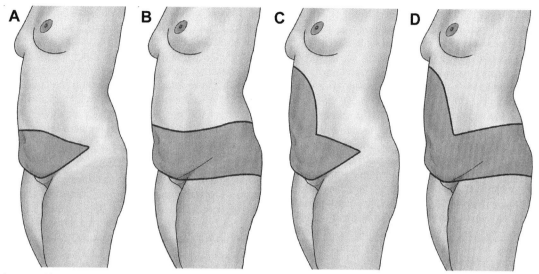

Fig. 5. Different approaches for lower body readjustment. (*A*) Anterior transverse (conventional), (*B*) circumferential (belt), (*C*) anterior combined (fleur-de-lis), and (*D*) circumferential combined (fleur-de-lis + belt).

post–bariatric surgery patients (**Fig. 5**C). This technique is mainly indicated for central pattern patients, whereby fat is deposited above the waistline and significantly expands the whole abdominal circumference. Because these cases generally do not present excess tissue or notable fallen lateral and posterior structures of the lower body, a combined anterior approach can provide better adjustment of the body contours by taking into account the recommended vectors for the required correction.

It is important to remember that although this technique can greatly improve contouring, it also leaves a visible and permanent median scar. It is up to the medical team to provide patients with detailed information about the pros and cons involved in this type of approach so they will collaborate in their surgical planning.

Combined Circumferential Approach

This technique also combines an anterior longitudinal resection with the circumferential approach specifically to address horizontal excess abdominal tissue, which is typically present in the post–bariatric surgery population (**Fig. 5**D). It is indicated for MWL patients with previous peripheral obesity and significant lower body deflation (below the waistline), but which also present some extent of central body circumferential laxity. Besides lifting lateral and posterior structures of the lower body, the combination with an anterior longitudinal resection can provide a tightening effect on the central body with the best contouring readjustment, by applying the most synergic vectors for

the necessary corrections. It is also important to consider the visible and permanent median scar that results from this procedure. The patients should be very well informed about the limitations and possibilities of each approach in order to actively cooperate toward the best surgical planning with an acceptable contour/scar ratio.

INNER SCAR UMBILICUS AND VERTICAL ABDOMINOPLASTY

Normal umbilical appearance is fundamental in order to achieve harmonious body contouring with aesthetically balanced abdominal results. The navel has been stated as the *surgeon's signature* and must receive appropriate attention during the abdominal approach, as no surgical outcome will be considered completely favorable if it presents with problems regarding shape, size, position, and scaring.[12–16] One important concept while managing the umbilicus is to keep in mind its anatomic landmarks, which include the base (a portion of abdominal skin closely attached to the rectus sheet), the grooving (circular skin wall between the deep base and superficial abdominal tissue), and the ring (rounded aspect of the abdominal skin that reflects into the grooving).

In the past decades, several investigators have recognized the hazards of outer umbilical scars in regular abdominoplasties, suggesting the complete amputation of the original stalk followed by different neo-umbilicoplasty techniques, promoting some kind of abdominal skin retraction into the deep rectus sheath.[17–21] In regular outer scar techniques, the incidence of necrosis, infection, and poor scaring may cause important distortions, ultimately with umbilical widening or stenosis, both conditions very difficult to deal with. Patients with MWL usually have long umbilical stalks, whose aponeurosis fixation ends up bulky and much more difficult to promote deep skin retraction. Shortening of the umbilical pedicle has been described but usually leads to a reduced skin area with poor scaring and subsequent umbilical stenosis.[5] In addition to that, such large tissue resections, usually required for body contouring in those patients, may produce intense traction vectors that might affect outer umbilical scars, leading to shape distortions. Especially for post–bariatric patients, when vertical abdominoplasty is indicated, preserving the original umbilicus stalk may increase those possible complications, related to the outer scar techniques.

Rebuilding umbilical architecture following abdominoplasty is considered one of the most challenging tasks, especially for patients with MWL who usually present with elongated umbilical stalks and critical tissue excess in both vertical and horizontal planes. Although anterior vertical resections may provide enhanced lower body contouring for that population, such indications have been restricted by visible and pathologic scaring usually with stigmatizing umbilical results. The presence of an outer scar around the umbilicus has been recognized as a source of several surgical complications that may lead to undesirable scaring with anatomic disarrangement and poor aesthetic results, ultimately figured by stenosis or widening of the navel.[4]

Franco and colleagues[22] introduced double lateral skin flaps to reconstruct the umbilicus within an anterior vertical scar, whereas several other investigators have also suggested similar approaches for creating a new umbilicus during the fleur-the-lis abdominoplasty.[23–29] Donnabella[28] popularized such a concept stating the importance of recreating all the umbilical anatomic landmarks (base, grooving, and ring) in search of natural results. Although conceptually comprehensive, those publications do not standardize and fully describe technical steps. Following those principles, the authors have suggested a specific and reproducible looping suture technique in order to anatomically recreate the new umbilicus.

Selection of Patients

The new inner scar umbilicoplasty may be indicated for patients of both sexes submitted to vertical abdominoplasties, with or without associated circumferential resections. Post–bariatric surgery patients should have a maximum body mass index

of 30 and present weight stabilization, which is defined in the authors' service by a variation inferior to 3% of the initial weight, within a 3-month period, whose verification begins at least 18 months after bariatric surgery.[30] Patients receive all the information regarding medical procedures, including aesthetic possibilities and limitations of the results, extensively described and accepted within the informed consent terms.

Markings

After midline and axillary lines demarcation, the authors place patients in the supine position to make a great upward traction of the abdominal tissue and then start the lower horizontal marking 5 cm above the vulvar commissure. With patients standing again, the authors laterally continue the inferior horizontal line toward both flanks, usually until around the midaxillary line projection. Anteriorly, they start the burying test to determine the transversal extent of the vertical resection. This maneuver consists of pushing the medial palm of one hand onto the anterior midline while the other hand equally grasps and moves both lateral tissue medially against each other and over the fixed midline. Burying midline tissue is an efficient way to make sure that lateral borders will successfully and safely close after its surgical resection. The lower level of the vertical resection is usually placed around the umbilicus, established by vigorous palpation of the flaps defining the turning point to start the upper horizontal marking, laterally to meet the ends of the previous lower lines.

Both vertical markings of the anterior resection include the design of the umbilical lateral skin flap, 8.0 cm wide × 1.5 cm long, that will be undermined and preserved by its pedicle, apart from the resected surgical specimen. The authors prefer to mark those lateral skin flaps initially wider than they will finally stand in order to allow a greater range of possibilities for better establishing the umbilical final position within the vertical scar, after moving and approximating the remaining abdominal flaps.[23]

Technique

In the supine position, the authors start the abdominal undermining through the inferior horizontal incision facing upwards until the umbilical level. After complete skin incision of the right vertical limb and flap elevation in both sides, cautery dissection is performed all the way through the subcutaneous tissue until the rectus sheath dissection plane. The same procedure on the left side joined both dissections at the vertical midline. During anterior tissue detachment, patients have

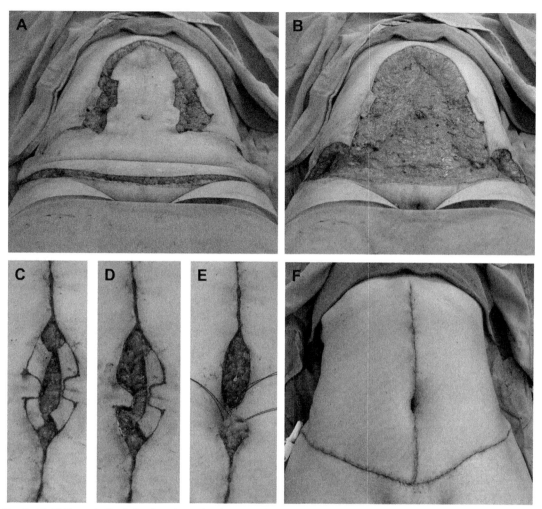

Fig. 6. (*A, B*) Fleur-de-lis abdominoplasty. (*C–E*) Neo-umbilicoplasty. Lateral flaps design, construction, and suture. (*F*) Final result.

the umbilical stalk isolated, clamped, and cut at its base, being finally resected along with the surgical specimen (**Fig. 6**A, B). A continuous closure suture with 2.0 nylon is performed at the amputated base just adjacent to the rectus sheath. Aponeurosis plication is performed as usual, whenever necessary. While suturing the vertical edges, both parallel skin flaps (8.0 cm wide × 1.5 cm long), preserved by the fleur-de-lis preoperative demarcation, are now intraoperatively redesigned into a proper size and position, at the iliac crest level, finally measuring approximately 2.5 × 1.5 cm (**Fig. 6**C–E). Rather than rectangular with sharp edges, the final shape of the flaps take a rounded design.[28] After removing excessive tissue and defatting the skin flaps, 3 nylon 3.0 sutures are placed in a looping technique in order to create a medial deep aponeurotic attachment, reconstructing the navel base (**Fig. 6**F).

Umbilical base: looping suture

(1) The looping suture needle initially enters the skin and transects the left flap exiting through the dermis, at 1.0 cm far from its edge. (2) It now enters the rectus sheet at the same side and runs immediately under it for 1.0 cm until exiting at the midline. (3) Then, the suture needle grasps 0.5 cm of the contralateral flap dermis exiting on its edge to perform the same 0.5 cm grasping on the left side, entering at its edge and exiting inside the dermal aspect of the flap. (4) The needle reenters the rectus sheet at the midline and runs immediately under it for 1.0 cm until exiting at the right side. (5) Finally, the needle transects the right flap entering the dermis and exiting throughout the skin, at 1.0 cm far from its edge. **Fig. 7** shows a schematic sequence of the umbilical base reconstruction by the lateral skin flaps.

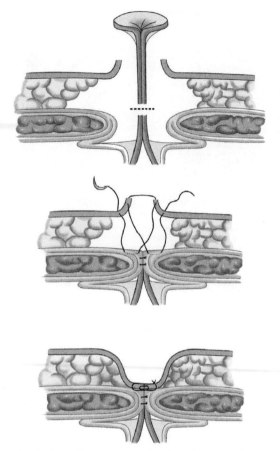

Fig. 7. Operative sequence showing stalk amputation and the looping sutures for neo-umbilicoplasty.

Three looping sutures are performed as mentioned earlier, one at the center and 2 others at the superior and inferior borders of the skin flaps. Initial stiches are left loose in order to facilitate the accomplishment of the following ones, and they are all progressively tightened at the end. This maneuver gradually helps to squeeze

the flaps against each other into the deep midline aponeurosis (**Fig. 8**).

Umbilical grooving: fat suture
Because it is not possible to retract the umbilical base deeper than the aponeurosis level, the best umbilical grooving will be achieved by increasing the projection of the surrounding areas. That is accomplished by two 2.0 polyglactin 910 (Vicryl, Ethicon Inc, Somerville, NJ) sutures, with a long needle (4 cm), approximating lateral fat tissue into the midline right above and immediately under the reconstructed umbilical base.

Umbilical ring
After reconstructing the base and establishing proper navel grooving, the 3-plane suture of the vertical edges helps to provide the ring configuration of the umbilicus, as it approximates the covering tissue under and above the new navel. After all, deeply cutaneous attachment to the rectus sheet (base) surrounded by normal subcutaneous tissue (grooving) and outer scarless skin configure the natural ring appearance to the surface of the abdominal wall around the umbilicus.

Fig. 8 shows a sequence of the intraoperative and immediate postoperative flap constitution. The skinapponeurotic looping suture makes it simple to accomplish the desired effect of squeezing the flaps against each other into the deep aponeurosis, in a most predictable maneuver.[10] The authors also prefer to use monofilament nylon sutures, which will be removed later, to avoid subcutaneous inflammatory reactions at the thin skin base. The authors found that maintaining loose external stiches to get them tightened only after completing all the looping passes not only facilitates the maneuvers but also makes them much more accurate and predictable than internal dermoaponeurotic suturing. The looping stiches are kept in place until completely removed after

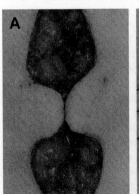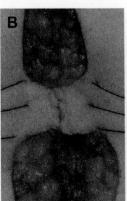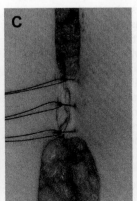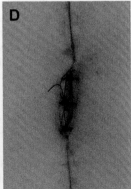

Fig. 8. Neo-umbilicoplasty: (*A*) lateral skin flaps; (*B, C*) the looping sutures; (*D*) final result.

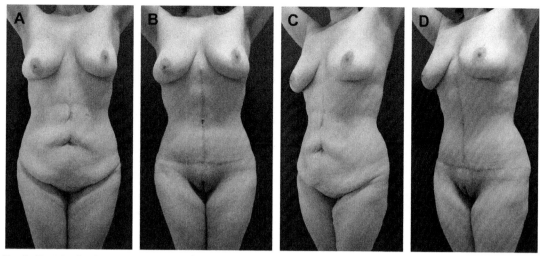

Fig. 9. Post–bariatric surgery patient who lost 45 kg, aged 23 years, with a body mass index of 27 kg/m², who underwent a fleur-de-lis procedure. (*A, C*) Preoperatively. (*B, D*) Eight months postoperatively.

30 days, whereas the horizontal and vertical limbs have absorbable internal sutures.

DISCUSSION

The post–bariatric surgery readjustment concept includes lifting and tightening of circumferential deflated tissue. Specifically on the central body, anterior longitudinal resections may help to provide the best contouring shapes; but visible resulting vertical scars have prevented patients and doctors to widely indicate such a procedure. In the same way, regular umbilical healing complications may lead to an unpleasant and stigmatizing abdominal aspect. The authors think that the inner scar umbilicus plays an important role in aesthetic enhancement of vertical approaches.

Figs. 9–12 show examples of natural and attractive postoperative results after fleur-de-lis abdominoplasties with and without circumferential belt lipectomy.

Aspiration drains are used in all cases for 5 to 10 days, until the daily debit drops to less than 40 mL. Prophylactic antibiotics are initiated intravenously in the operating room (30 minutes before the incision) and maintained orally for several days after hospital discharge. The authors have previously presented a series of 110 consecutive patients[30]; the most common complications of vertical abdominoplasties include small spots of dehiscence along the suture lines and seromas, both conservatively treated. The authors had no cases of infection, skin necrosis, or thromboembolic events.

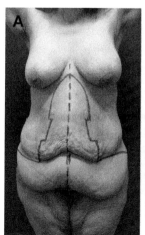
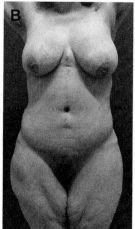
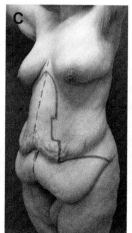
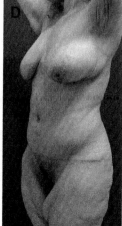

Fig. 10. Post–bariatric surgery patient who lost 72 kg, aged 31 years, with a body mass index of 28 kg/m², who underwent a fleur-de-lis procedure. (*A, C*) Preoperatively. (*B, D*) Twelve months postoperatively.

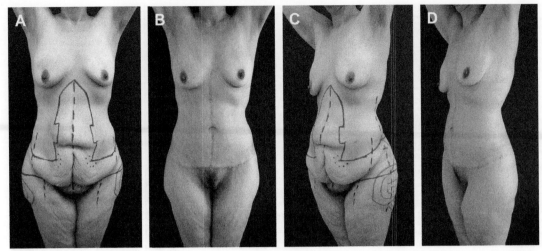

Fig. 11. Post–bariatric surgery patient who lost 50 kg, aged 35 years, with a body mass index of 26 kg/m², who underwent a circumferential (belt) + fleur-de-lis procedure. (*A, C*) Preoperatively. (*B, D*) Ten months postoperatively.

It is interesting to note that individuals present several different umbilical shapes, but all of them may be considered normal as long as their anatomic landmarks are well defined (base, grooving, and ring). After birth, a central skin retraction is responsible to create the umbilical anatomy, and the most natural surgical reconstruction will be achieved by procedures that best reproduce such a physiologic healing process. Although the authors' inner scar umbilicus technique is well defined and equally performed with standard maneuvers, the resulting umbilical shapes usually vary, even with keeping the mentioned anatomic landmarks (**Fig. 13**). Skin quality, subcutaneous thickness, and scar retraction are some of the variables that may influence the final navel aspect, just like it happens in nature, whereby several different umbilical shapes might develop to be considered normal, both in men and women. The lack of external scaring and the inner healing pattern of the new umbilicus also seem to help establish better scar quality for both superior and inferior abdominal vertical scars.

Patients quite commonly present with a mild inflammatory exudate arising from the new umbilicus during the initial 15 to 20 days, with total

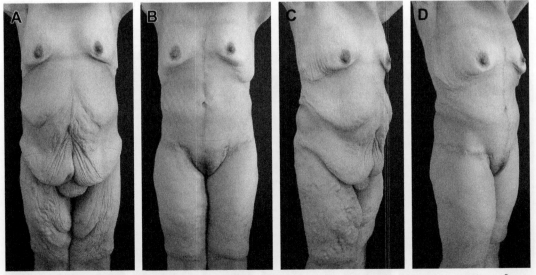

Fig. 12. Post–bariatric surgery patient who lost 80 kg, aged 38 years, with a body mass index of 26 kg/m², who underwent a circumferential (belt) + fleur-de-lis procedure. (*A, C*) Preoperatively. (*B, D*) Eighteen months postoperatively + internal vertical thigh reduction (6 months postoperatively).

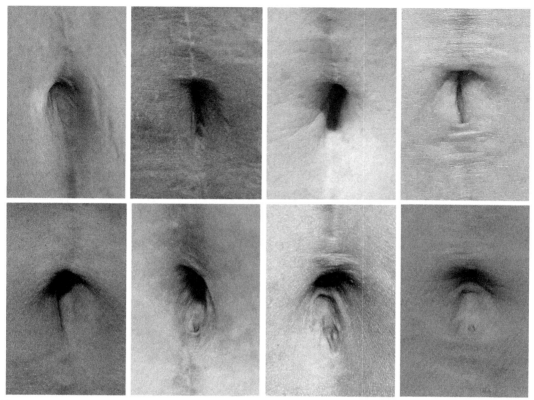

Fig. 13. Neo-umbilicoplasty. Natural results with different shapes, keeping normal anatomic landmarks.

resolution by conservative open and dry dressings. The authors have not reported any further umbilical complications, such as infection, necrosis, dehiscence, widening, or stenosis. Patients usually show natural and scarless new navels with nice shapes and proper position.

The inner scar umbilicus is a simple, safe, and reproducible technique, presenting low complication rates with sustainable, nice, and natural results. The high quality of navel tridimensional reconstruction makes it the authors' first choice for vertical abdominoplasties and favors its indication, especially for post–bariatric surgery body contouring.

REFERENCES

1. Wolf AM, Boioiogol U. The effect of loss of excess weight on the metabolic risk factors after bariatric surgery in morbidly and super-obese patients. Obes Surg 2007;17:910–9.
2. Agha Mohammadi S, Hurwitz DJ. Potential impacts of nutritional deficiency of postbariatric patients on body contouring surgery. Plast Reconstr Surg 2008;122:1901–14.
3. Pinho PR, Chillof CLM, Mendes FH, et al. Psychological approach for post-bariatric plastic surgery. Rev Bras Cir Plast 2011;26(4):685–90.
4. Mendes FH, Viterbo F. Abdominoplasty after massive weight loss. In: Avelar JM, editor. New concepts on abdominoplasties and further applications, Switzerland: Springer; 2016. p. 356–8.
5. Mendes FH, Viterbo F, editors. Cirurgia Plastica Pós Bariátrica. Rio de Janeiro (Brazil): DiLivros; 2016.
6. Markman B, Barton F Jr. Anatomy of the subcutaneous tissue of the trunk and lower extremities. Plast Reconstr Surg 1980;80:248.
7. Avelar J. Regional distribution and behaviour of the subcutaneous tissue concerning selection and indication for liposuction. Aesthetic Plast Surg 1989;13: 155.
8. Lockwood TE. Superficial fascial system (SFS) of the trunk and extremities: a new concept. Plast Reconstr Surg 1991;87:1009–18.
9. Aly AS. Belt lipectomy. In: Aly AS, editor. Body contouring after massive weight loss. St Louis (MO): Quality Medical; 2006. p. 71–145.
10. Rahban SR, Gross JE. A new approach to correction of truncal redundancy after massive weight loss – the lateral thoracoabdominoplasty. Aesthetic Surg J 2007;27:518–23.
11. Modolin M, Cintra W Jr, Gobbi CI, et al. Circumferential abdominoplasty for sequential treatment after morbid obesity. Obes Surg 2003;13:95–100.
12. Baroudi R. Umbilicoplasty. Clin Plast Surg 1975;2: 431–48.

13. Juri J, Juri C, Raiden G. Reconstruction of the umbilicus in abdominoplasty. Plast Reconstr Surg 1979; 63:580–2.

14. Malic CC, Spyrou GE, Hough M, et al. Patient satisfaction with two different methods of umbilicoplasty. Plast Reconstr Surg 2007;119:357–61.

15. Craig SB, Faller MS, Puckett CL. In search of the ideal female umbilicus. Plast Reconstr Surg 2000; 105:389–92.

16. Rohrich RJ, Sorokin ES, Brown SA, et al. Is the umbilicus truly midline? Clinical and medicolegal implications. Plast Reconstr Surg 2003;112:259–63.

17. Illouz YG. A new safe and aesthetic approach to suction abdominoplasty. Aesthetic Plast Surg 1992; 16:237–45.

18. Clo TCT. Neoomphaloplasty using an X-shaped incision in 401 consecutive abdominoplasties. Rev Bras Cir Plást 2013;28(3):375–80.

19. Nogueira DSC. Routine neoomphaloplasty during abdominoplasties. Rev Bras Cir Plást 2008;23(3): 207–13.

20. Freitas JOG, Guerreiro V, Sperli AE. Neoonphaloplasty in abdominal dermolipectomy: double "V" technique. Rev Bras Cir Plast 2010;25(3):504–8.

21. Abreu Ng JA. Abdominoplasty: neo omphaloplasty without scar or fat excision. Rev Bras Cir Plast 2010;25(3):499–503.

22. Franco D, Medeiros J, Farias C, et al. Umbilical reconstruction for patients with a midline scar. Aesthetic Plast Surg 2006;30(5):595–8.

23. Silva FN, Oliveira EA. Neoonphaloplasty in vertical abdominoplasty. Rev Bras Cir Plast 2010;25:330–6.

24. Reno AB, Mizukami A, Calaes IL, et al. Neoomphaloplasty in anchor-line abdominoplasty performed in patients who have previously undergone bariatric surgery. Rev Bras Cir Plast 2013;28(1):114–8.

25. Cavalcante ELF. Neo-umbilicoplasty as an option in umbilical reconstruction in abdominal anchor dermolipectomy post gastroplasty. Rev Bras Cir Plast 2010;25(3):509–18.

26. Monte ALR. Treatment of the umbilical stenosis in a vertical dermolipectomy patient. Rev Bras Cir Plast 2011;26(1):167–70.

27. Mizukami A, Ribeiro BB, Reno BA, et al. Retrospective analysis of 70 patients who underwent post-bariatric abdominoplasty with neo-omphaloplasty. Rev Bras Cir Plast 2014;29(1):89–93.

28. Donnabella A. Anatomical reconstruction of the umbilicus. Rev Bras Cir Plást 2013;28:119–23.

29. Mendes FH, Viterbo F. Inner scar umbilicus: new horizons for vertical abdominoplasty. Plast Reconstr Surg 2018;141(4):507e–16e.

30. Mendes FH, Viterbo F. Defining weight stability for post bariatric body contouring procedures. Aesthetic Plast Surg 2017;41:979–80.

Buttock Lifting
The Golden Rules

Check for updates

Jean-Francois Pascal, MD

KEYWORDS

- Buttock lift • Tightening rule • Cutting principles • Volume • Violin deformation • Skin excess
- Buttock volume • Buttock augmentation • Buttock fat flap

KEY POINTS

- To be successful with a body lift, it is mandatory to know the differences of tissue quality at the back area and respect the rules of 16 and 4; this is the only way to avoid complications and to get an enthusiastic result.
- It can make a significant contribution to quality of life, especially in massive weight loss patients.
- Thanks to this new technique, the lower body lift has now become a much more reliable and effective surgical procedure.

INTRODUCTION

After 30 years of buttocks surgery, especially after massive weight loss, a series of more than 800 cases and a thesis in 2010, the author became convinced about some precise rules. According to him, the failure to observe these rules will lead to poor results or complications.

The goal of this article is to demonstrate that buttock lifting requires precise knowledge and technique.

WHY BUTTOCKS AESTHETIC IS SO IMPORTANT?

In primates, who are quadruped, the posterior area has an essential role; it allows reproduction and species survival. This area, in human ancestors, sent many sexual signals and allowed optimizing fertilization. As a legacy from the past, human beings get a strong and animal attraction for buttocks. At the end, there is understanding why aesthetics of buttocks are so important and why the demand is so big.[1–3]

THE IDEAL BUTTOCK

The goal of the surgery is to recreate an ideal buttock (**Fig. 1**). The volume is variable depending on ethnic groups, but the basic data of the ideal buttocks are precise.

The ideal buttock is: round, with a firm look, equally long as it is wide, with a smooth surface, highly positioned with a short infrabuttock fold. The areas up to the buttocks are also essential to buttock definition. Flanks must be flat or curved.

A recent study from University of Texas at Austin clarifies on another standard of beauty. The study, published in *Evolution and Human Behavior* in 2015, shows that the male brain is programmed to favor women with a curvy backside with a 45.5° from the back to the buttocks. This dates to prehistoric influences. The explanation is that 45.5° angle of lumbar curvature allowed ancestral women to better support, provide for, and carry out multiple pregnancies.[4–10]

CONSEQUENCES OF THE SKIN EXCESS

Damage of the elastic and collagen fibers related to skin excess may occur with classical factors: genetically bad skin quality, aging process, and small or massive weight losses (**Fig. 2**).

Skin damage is even worse when there is significant loss of volume.

Patients complains about:

- Too soft and mobile buttocks, especially when they exercise

---

The author has nothing to disclose.
Head of Scientific Council, IPSAC, 8 Quai Général Sarrail, Lyon 69006, France
E-mail address: jfpascal69@gmail.com

Clin Plastic Surg 46 (2019) 61–70
https://doi.org/10.1016/j.cps.2018.08.008

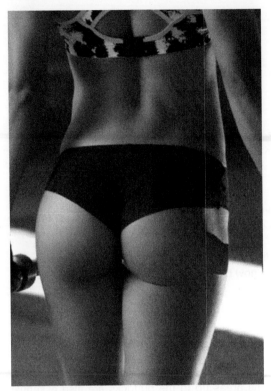

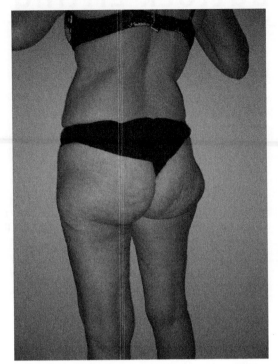

Fig. 2. Buttock damage caused by the aging process: dimples, shape damage, interbuttock fold lengthening.

Fig. 1. The ideal buttock is: round, with a firm look, as long as it is wide, with a smooth surface, highly positioned with a short infrabuttock fold. Flanks must be flat or curved with a 45.5° degree lumbar curvature from the back to the buttocks.

- Sagging
- Infrabuttock fold lengthening
- Shape damage, mainly flattening
- Irregularities of the surface, often mistaken with cellulitis
- Waves at the lower buttocks[11–13]

THE TIGHTENING RULE OF 16

It is essential to understand this rule to understand the drawings. Skin is elastic and absorbs tension. This means that there is no force transmitted further than 16 cm from the scar line. This rule works for the entire body. For example, that is why, at the lateral thigh, it is not possible to correct lower than 16 cm with a cutting at the beltline (**Fig. 3**). And that is why, for a perfect buttock tightening, the drawing is located at 16 cm up from the infrabuttock fold. Therefore, most buttock lifting procedures are not efficient enough: because of a too high located skin resection. Surgeons often locate it following a gull-wing shape up to the buttock volume. The gull-wing shape is beautiful but not efficient for buttock lifting. In other words,

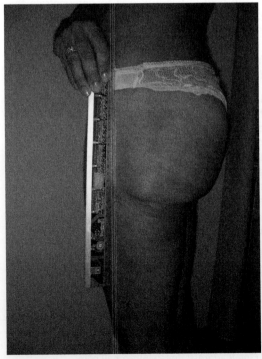

Fig. 3. Tightening rule of 16: no stretching lower than 16 cm.

to be efficient, the resection band must be horizontal and based low. This is my tightening rule of 16.

ANALYSIS OF THE DIFFERENT AREAS AT THE BUTTOCKS

At the posterior part of the body (**Fig. 4**), there are 4 different areas that require a different approach:

- Interbuttock fold: skin is stuck to the bone, has a poor mobility and the sitting position making high demands on it; consequently, wound dehiscence is frequent and can be large, especially at the beginning of the learning curve (**Fig. 5**); no undermining up or down is allowed in this area because of the richness in lymphatic trunks
- Buttocks: if the skin is much softer, then the resection width will be bigger; undermining is possible, because the area is poor in lymphatic trunks
- Lateral thigh: if the skin is more rigid then the resection width is reduced; in the case of bad tissues or too much tension, the fat will tear following with violin deformation (described later)

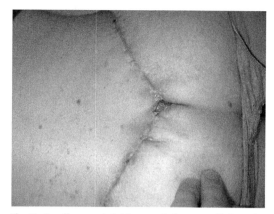

Fig. 5. Small wound dehiscence is frequent if the rules are not respected: no undermining, skin resection superficial, rule of 4.

- Lateral line: it separates the front and the back part of the body; at the front, tissues are pulled down; at the back, tissues are raised (in female body lift); then, it is a problem to get a horizontal scar line at the transition zone

MARKINGS

Precise markings are essential for many aspects.[14–18] They ensure the right resection width, the symmetry of the tightening, and the scar positioning. The resection should be low in women and high in men, but the main point is the blood conservation. Accurate drawing allows the injection of epinephrine at the beginning of the procedure to the correct areas. After allowing the epinephrine to work (15 minutes), the procedure is essentially bloodless.

The markings are based on the rules of 16: point and line (**Fig. 6**). This rule is essential and

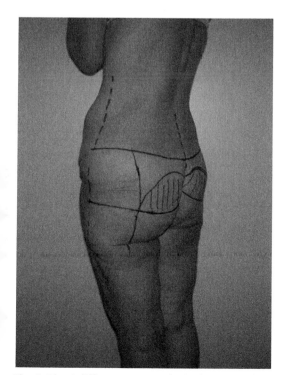

Fig. 4. The 4 different areas at the back. Interbuttock fold, buttock (area with the flap), vertical line of 16, lateral line.

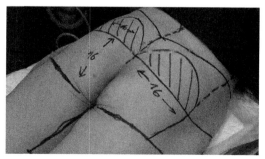

Fig. 6. The 3 rules of 16: distance from the lower incision line to the infrabuttock fold drawn in the lying position, distance from the posterior line to the of 16 drawn in the standing position, LP flap width.

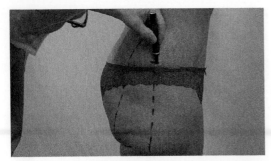

Fig. 7. Laterally, the upper incision point is located slightly up to the underwear line to anticipate a lowering caused by the tension of closure.

it is important to understand, and the operation will be suboptimal if the rules of 16 are not respected:

- I begin the drawing laterally and in standing position. I draw the upper incision point, which is located slightly up to the underwear line (**Fig. 7**) to anticipate a lowering caused by the tension of the closure. At the end, the scar line will be perfectly hidden under the underwear. Then I perform the first pinch test to place the lower incision point.
- I carry on in lying position at the interbuttock fold. Here I begin with the lower incision point located at 16 cm from the infrabuttock fold (point of 16). The goal is to avoid lengthening the interbuttock fold, which is ugly but frequent. Therefore, in many massive weight loss patients, there will be a interbuttock fold resection to maintain it at a normal size. Starting from this point, I perform a pinch test to

estimate the resection width, and I mark the upper incision point.
- Then I mark the superior horizontal cutting line by gently pulling down and joining the posterior and lateral dots.
- The inferior cutting line (**Fig. 8**) is a little more complicated to draw, and I must introduce a new vertical line: the line of 16. These 16 cm are of course an average, and this vertical line can oscillate between 14 and 17 depending on the body width. It is drawn in the standing position. This line separates the buttock and the lateral thigh area. If you look closer, you will notice that the skin quality is totally different. At the buttock area, skin is loose. At the thigh area, skin is firmer. So, the skin resection will be obviously thinner laterally, and finally the lower incision line will be a curve.

At the buttock area (starting from the midline as far as the line of 16), the incision line is drawn horizontally and in lying position with gentle pulling up. It is drawn at 16 cm from the infrabuttock fold to respect the tightening rule. This is the only way to achieve a good tightening and to restore a high positioned buttock with a short infrabuttock fold. At the end of the operation, this distance will become 20 cm thanks to the closure tension.

Laterally, the inferior incision line rises to join the inferior lateral dot (**Fig. 9**).

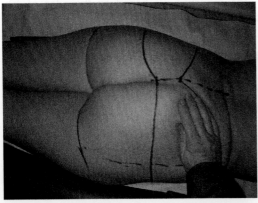

Fig. 8. The inferior cutting line is drawn horizontally and in the lying position with gentle pulling up. It is drawn at 16 cm from the infrabuttock fold to respect the tightening rule.

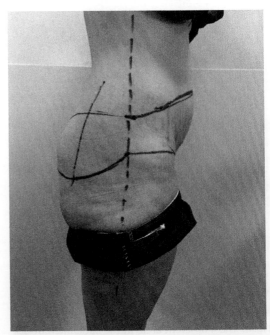

Fig. 9. Laterally, the inferior incision line rises to join the inferior lateral dot.

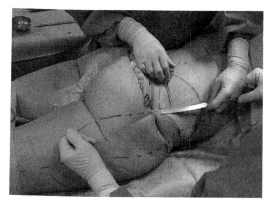

Fig. 10. Rule of 4: The right tension of closure is the one that leaves a play of the tissue of 4 cm. The forceps show the remaining tissue laxity while pulling down.

At the end, there are 2 precise cutting lines ready to be injected.

To sum up, the consequences of not respecting the rule of 16 are catastrophic for female body lift:

- Less efficient tightening at the lower buttock
- Infrabuttock fold shortening less efficient
- Interbuttock fold and buttock lengthening
- LP flap (Le Louarn and Pascal flap for autoaugmentation) too highly located and not mobile
- High-lying scar impossible to hide wearing low-rise jeans

At the front, in case of a 360° body lift, the markings are a little bit different from a regular abdominoplasty. In a regular abdominoplasty, the lower incision line follows the same direction as the inguinal fold to avoid going out of the underwear. In a body lift, the lower incision line crosses the

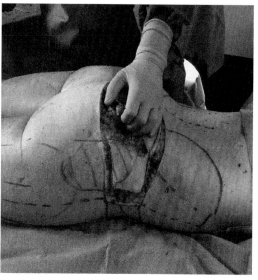

Fig. 12. P flap. The P flap is useful to avoid the violin deformation. The flap size is designed depending on the need to fill the lateral space. As for the LP flap, the skin of the P flap is totally resected. I only keep a part of the lateral tissues that are normally removed. I plan the size to avoid creating a visible lateral bump. If the flap is too big, it is possible to reduce it in supine position. Most of the time, I create a small pocket downwards to better spread the volume, and I anchor at the lower pocket with 1 or 2 sutures.

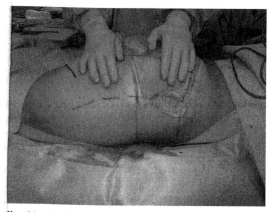

Fig. 11. At the lateral area, it is essential to begin with the upper line to avoid the lowering of the scar, which becomes visible outside the underwear. The reduction of drawing will come from the lower line.

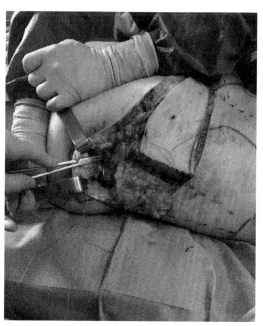

Fig. 13. P flap. Skin has been removed. Pocket has been created downwards, and I am placing 1 suture.

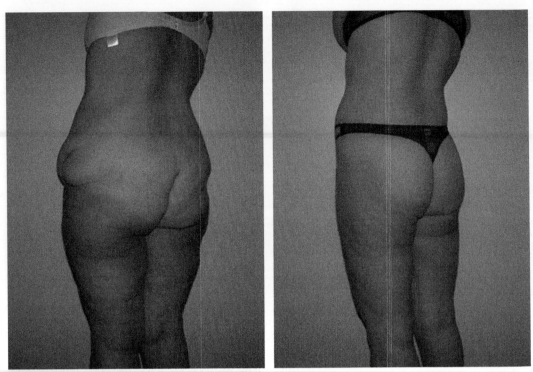

Fig. 14. 26-year-old patient after a 80 kg massive weight loss. Dramatic improvement of the buttock shape with LP flap.

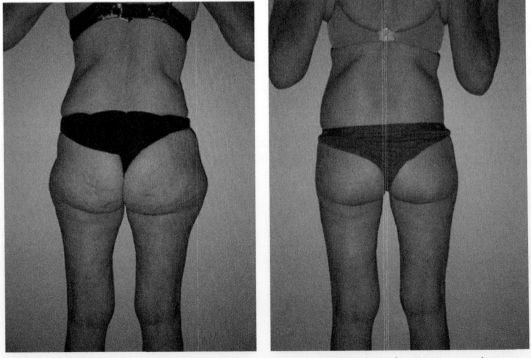

Fig. 15. Aging process with a strong damage at the buttock and lateral thigh. Perfect improvement because of the respect of the tightening rules.

inguinal fold, because all the tissues of the anterior thigh will rise after closing and finally will be included underneath the underwear.

CUTTING PRINCIPLES: THE RULE OF 4

The goals of these principles are to control and secure the skin resection (**Fig. 10**). There are many questions that must be answered before cutting:

- Will you be able to close if you cut all at once ?
- If you manage to close, are you sure to close with the right tension (the one which produces no wound dehiscence and good quality scar)?

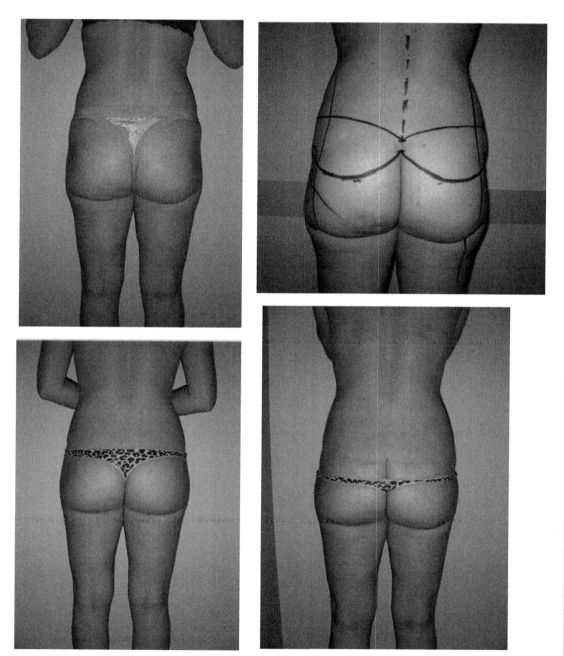

Fig. 16. In this case, the goal was to reduce the buttock height and the volume. The rejuvenation is big. The scar, after 1 year, is well located and of good quality.

- When cutting, do you begin with the lower incision line or the upper one?
- If you must modify the drawing, will you move the upper line or the lower one?

The drawing is just an estimation of the resection width, because there are many sources of error while performing it (eg, tissue elasticity, strength of the hand pulling, body shape), so it is not possible to cut all at once and pray if you will be able to close and with what tension.

The right tension of closure is the one that leaves a play of the tissue of 4 cm. It is essential to leave 4 cm of extra tissue, because tissues are fragile; additionally, too much tension will lead to fat necrosis and wound dehiscence. This is the rule of 4.

The intraoperative technique to leave 4 cm skin laxity is easy to perform with a thread.

About the cutting sequence

- The best way is to begin cutting with the lower line at the buttock area to be sure to respect the rule of 16 and get a perfect tightening. If there is a reduction of the drawing, it will come from the upper part.
- At the lateral area, it is essential to begin with the upper line to avoid the lowering of the scar, which becomes visible outside the underwear. The reduction of drawing will come from the lower line (**Fig. 11**).

ABOUT BUTTOCK VOLUME

Buttock lifting inevitably reduces the buttock volume. Then, there are 3 different situations:

- Reduction is required, because the buttocks are too big.
- The patient would like a preservation of the volume only. Then, I use the LP flap.
- The patient would like a volume augmentation. Then I often use 3 techniques depending on the case: LP flap, lipofilling, or implant.

About LP Flap (Le Louarn and Pascal's Flap)

Le Louarn and I published the LP flap in 2002.[19–22] Later, many authors published their flap. They all share an elevation of the flap to better mobilize it. I think that it is risky, and I totally discourage undermining the flap. In fact, this elevation becomes necessary, because the flap is too highly designed in the fat of the flank (in fact the whole drawing is too high). The flap must be designed low in the fat of the buttocks to fill the buttock. As this fat is mobile, there is no need to elevate it.

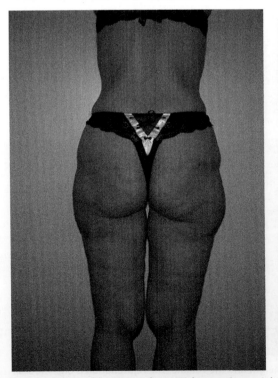
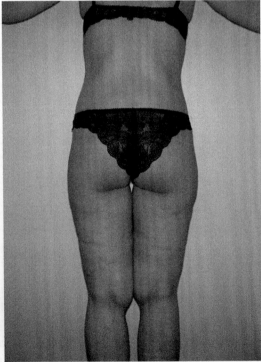

Fig. 17. 45-year-old patient after a 50 kg massive weight loss. Buttock and thigh lifting.

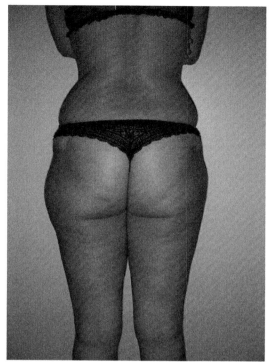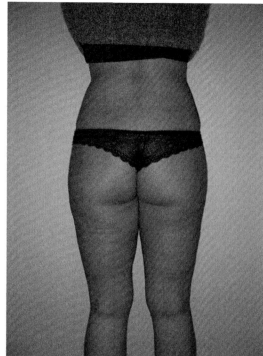

Fig. 18. No weight loss but congenital gynoid body shape. Perfect reshaping.

About the New P flap (Pascal's Flap)

The P flap is a new island flap located laterally to the LP flap (**Figs. 12** and **13**).[23–25] I created it to avoid the frequent violin deformation caused by the tearing of the fat underneath the scar line at the lateral thigh. I use it in 90% of my 360° body lifts, especially if tissues are heavy. The flap size is designed depending on the need to fill the lateral space. As for the LP flap, the skin of the P flap is totally resected. I only keep a part of the lateral tissues that are normally removed. I plan the size to avoid creating a visible lateral bump. If the flap is too big, it is possible to reduce it in the supine position. Most of the time, I create a small pocket downwards to better spread the volume, and I anchor the flap at the lower pocket with 1 or t2 sutures.

SUMMARY

To be successful with a body lift, it is mandatory to know the differences of tissue quality at the back area and respect the rules of 16 and 4. This is the only way to avoid complications and to get an enthusiastic result (**Figs. 14–18**). The outcomes are spectacular every time. It can make a significant contribution to quality of life, especially in massive weight loss patients. Thanks to this new technique, the lower body lift has now become a much more reliable and effective surgical procedure.

REFERENCES

1. Raynal P, Le Meaux JP, Chereau E. Anthropologic evolution of women's pelvis. Gynecol Obstet Fertil 2005;33(7–8):464–8.
2. Montagu A. The buttocks and natural selection. JAMA 1966;198(1):169.
3. Schwartz MB, Brownell KD. Obesity and body image. Body Image 2004;1(1):43–56.
4. Mendieta CG. Classification system for gluteal evaluation. Clin Plast Surg 2006;33(3):333–46.
5. Cuenca-Guerra R, Quezada J. What makes buttocks beautiful? A review and classification of the determinants of gluteal beauty and the surgical techniques to achieve them. Aesthetic Plast Surg 2004;28(5):340–7.
6. Centeno RF, Young VL. Clinical anatomy in aesthetic gluteal body contouring surgery. Clin Plast Surg 2006;33(3):347–58.
7. Cuenca-Guerra R, Lugo-Beltran I. Beautiful buttocks: characteristics and surgical techniques. Clin Plast Surg 2006;33(3):321–32.
8. Centeno RF. Gluteal aesthetic unit classification: a tool to improve outcomes in body contouring. Aesthet Surg J 2006;26(2):200–8.

9. Singh D. Ideal female body shape: role of body weight and waist-to-hip ratio. Int J Eat Disord 1994; 16(3):283–8.

10. Singh D. Female judgment of male attractiveness and desirability for relationships: role of waist-to-hip ratio and financial status. J Pers Soc Psychol 1995;69(6):1089–101.

11. Gonzalez R. Etiology, definition, and classification of gluteal ptosis. Aesthetic Plast Surg 2006;30(3):320–6.

12. Coleman WP 3rd. Autologous fat transplantation. Plast Reconstr Surg 1991;88(4):736.

13. Pascal JF, Le Louarn C. Remodeling bodylift with high lateral tension. Aesthetic Plast Surg 2002; 26(3):223–30.

14. Lockwood T. Lower body lift with superficial fascial system suspension. Plast Reconstr Surg 1993; 92(6):1112–22 [discussion: 1123–5].

15. Aly A, Cram A. The Iowa belt lipectomy technique. Plast Reconstr Surg 2008;122(3):959–60.

16. Jones BM, Toft NJ. Bodylifting: indications, technique and complications. J Plast Reconstr Aesthet Surg 2008;61(7):730–5.

17. Capella JF. Body lift. Clin Plast Surg 2008;35(1): 27–51 [discussion: 93].

18. Van Geertruyden JP, Vandeweyer E, de Fontaine S, et al. Circumferential torsoplasty. Br J Plast Surg 1999;52(8):623–8.

19. Sozer SO, Agullo FJ, Palladino H. Bilateral lumbar hip dermal fat rotation flaps: a novel technique for autologous augmentation gluteoplasty. Plast Reconstr Surg 2007;119(3):1126–7 [author reply: 7–8].

20. Rohde C, Gerut ZE. Augmentation buttock-pexy using autologous tissue following massive weight loss. Aesthet Surg J 2005;25(6):576–81.

21. Colwell AS, Borud LJ. Autologous gluteal augmentation after massive weight loss: aesthetic analysis and role of the superior gluteal artery perforator flap. Plast Reconstr Surg 2007;119(1): 345–56.

22. Raposo-Amaral CE, Cetrulo CL Jr, Guidi Mde C, et al. Bilateral lumbar hip dermal fat rotation flaps: a novel technique for autologous augmentation gluteoplasty. Plast Reconstr Surg 2006;117(6): 1781–8.

23. Pascal JF, Le Louarn C. Bodylift complications. Ann Chir Plast Esthet 2004;49(6):605–9.

24. Maladry D, Pascal JF. Outline surgery after massive weight loss or gastroplasty. Ann Chir Plast Esthet 2003;48(5):405–11.

25. Gisquet H, Pascal JF. le remodelage glutéal après perte de poids massive, thèse de médecine. Université NANCY; 2010.

Breast Reshaping After Massive Weight Loss

Omar E. Beidas, MD[a], J. Peter Rubin, MD[b],*

KEYWORDS

- Body contouring • Plastic surgery • Massive weight loss • Breast • Mastopexy
- Dermal suspension • Parenchymal reshaping

KEY POINTS

- The breasts of patients with massive weight loss cannot always be treated with traditional breast reshaping techniques because of the extent of the deformity.
- Patients should be screened according to the most up-to-date guidelines by the American Cancer Society.
- Dermal suspension, parenchymal reshaping mastopexy (DSPRM) can be safely combined with other body contouring procedures.
- DSPRM complications are minimal and generally easily treated on an outpatient basis.

INTRODUCTION

For years, plastic surgeons have been tasked with restoring the aged, ptotic breast to its youthful state.[1] Traditional mastopexy techniques focus on tightening the skin envelope by means of skin excision and minimal parenchymal dissection to raise the gland to a natural position on the chest wall. Perhaps in no other patient is a long-lasting, aesthetic result difficult to achieve than in patients with massive weight loss (MWL). This population presents with a characteristic deformity: a ptotic, deflated breast with medialized nipples and defined axillary roll.

The technique described herein was developed by the author after years of operating on these patients without achieving a desirable cosmetic result that stood the test of time. This novel procedure incorporates a combination of parenchymal reshaping, dermal suspension, and selective auto-augmentation. The operation, aptly termed a *dermal suspension, parenchymal reshaping mastopexy* (DSPRM), involves a stepwise correction of the breast deformity seen in the MWL population.

BREAST DEFORMITIES AFTER MASSIVE WEIGHT LOSS

Based on the position of the nipple and breast parenchyma relative to the inframammary fold (IMF), Regnault[2] classified ptosis into 3 stages. A natural, young breast has a nipple position projected at or above the level of the IMF with most of the breast tissue above the IMF. In first-degree ptosis, the nipple is within 1 cm of the anterior projection of the IMF. In second-degree ptosis, the nipple has descended to a point between 1 and 3 cm lower than the IMF. At this stage, the nipple still sits on the anterior projection of the breast mound, whereas in third-degree ptosis, the nipple rests on the most dependent portion of the breast. Finally, pseudoptosis describes a breast with a nipple that sits within 1 cm of the IMF but where most of the breast parenchyma has fallen below the fold.

The author has nothing to disclose.
[a] 3380 Boulevard of the Allies, Suite 180, Pittsburgh, PA 15213, USA; [b] 3550 Terrace Street, 6B Scaife Hall, Pittsburgh, PA 15261, USA
* Corresponding author.
E-mail address: rubipj@UPMC.EDU

Clin Plastic Surg 46 (2019) 71–76
https://doi.org/10.1016/j.cps.2018.08.009

plasticsurgery.theclinics.com

Although this staging system encompasses the typical aging breast, it does not consider the distinct deformities seen after MWL. The process of stretching the skin during weight gain followed by shrinking the parenchyma secondary to weight loss leaves a deflated, ptotic breast with poor skin envelope. There are 4 notable anatomic features, present in variable degrees, that characterize the female breast after MWL:

a. Significant breast volume loss, with deflation and flattening of the breast against the chest wall
b. Relative skin excess compared with parenchymal volume, along with loss of skin elasticity
c. Medialized nipple position
d. Prominent axillary roll that extends into or beyond the midaxillary line with loss of the lateral curve of the breast

PATIENT EVALUATION (INDICATIONS/CONTRAINDICATIONS)

Consideration must be paid to the characteristic breast deformities that appear in patients after MWL, including a flattened appearance secondary to loss of fatty tissue, significant skin excess with inelasticity, and a medialized nipple.[3] However, not all women present with these deformities after MWL. Each patient must be evaluated individually; based on the nipple position and estimated amount of tissue resection, the surgeon determines the method that will appropriately site the nipple and mold the parenchyma.

For those presenting with milder deformities, traditional techniques are generally adequate to reshape the breast.[4] In patients with minimal ptosis, a peri-areolar reduction mastopexy usually suffices. Moderate deformities generally require a vertical incision on the breast, whereas severe deformities dictate an inverted-T incision to excise both horizontal and vertical skin laxity. In patients presenting with the characteristic breast deformities listed earlier, traditional mastopexy techniques do not adequately address the problem. Rather, extensive procedures are required to restore an anatomic reshape to the breast, which entails a Wise-pattern DSPRM to treat the deflated, ptotic breast.[5,6]

Before surgery, patients should be optimized from a nutritional, medical, and psychological standpoint. Patients should undergo breast cancer screening according to the American Cancer Society's most recent guidelines.[7] DSPRM is safe to perform at the same time as other truncal or extremity contouring procedures, as demonstrated by a review of the author's experience with the MWL population.[8] In this series of 91 patients, 93.4% of patients underwent DSPRM combined

with abdominoplasty, upper or lower body lift, brachioplasty, thigh-plasty, or a combination thereof. Losken and Holtz's[6] experience with breast procedures showed that breast reshaping could be safely combined with other procedures as well. However, one must be careful when combining DSPRM with abdominal contouring procedures, as the truncal reshaping can shift the IMF. Therefore, the abdominal portion should be performed first to avoid postoperative distortion of the IMF. When performed simultaneously or at a separate time, the DSPRM incision can be blended nicely into a brachioplasty or upper body lift incision.

There are no true contraindications to this procedure if patients meet the anatomic criteria and are safe to undergo surgery. However, this technique should absolutely be avoided in active nicotine users because of the extensive undermining required for flap design. Furthermore, implants are not recommended in patients with MWL, as they are associated with additional complications, recurrent ptosis, and malposition, leading to increased rates of revision procedures.

SURGICAL TECHNIQUE
Markings

Breast meridians are marked bilaterally to identify the bisection of breast parenchyma on each hemichest. This new meridian will correct a medialized nipple position. A typical Wise pattern is marked centered on each meridian, with a lateral limb extending farther than usual to use as a dermoglandular pedicle that will volumize the lateral breast. Pictures of markings are shown in **Fig. 1**. This lateral axillary extension can be modified in length and width based on patients' unique anatomy; however, only tissue beyond the posterior axillary line should not be used in the auto-augmentation, as the blood supply to this region is not as reliable. Note that even if the excess tissue extends far posteriorly, only what is needed for auto-augmentation is used and the remainder is excised. If patients have undergone or plan to undergo a brachioplasty or upper body lift, those incisions can be blended nicely into the mastopexy incision. Described next is the dermal suspension technique that is commonly used for this patient population.[5]

Intraoperative Steps

A solution of 1:100,000 of epinephrine in normal saline is injected subcutaneously along the skin markings and into the regions of planned dissection. Intradermal injection can be used to hydrodissect the epidermis and decrease blood loss during de-epithelialization. Ideally, this should be

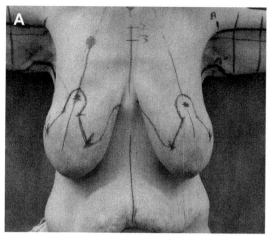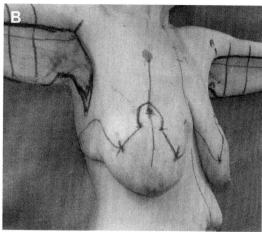

Fig. 1. Preoperative images of a patient marked for a dermal suspension, parenchymal reshaping procedure. (*A*) A Wise-pattern mastopexy is drawn on the chest centered on the breast meridian. (*B*) Note the lateral extension of the pattern along the chest wall. It is not recommended to include tissue posterior to the posterior axillary line in the pedicle; however, excess tissue in this zone can be resected.

allowed to instill for at least 10 minutes before an incision is made to allow the epinephrine time to take effect. To minimize inefficient use of operating room time, injection can be done off the field as soon as patients are asleep, before prepping and draping.

The nipple-areola complex (NAC) is marked with the surgeon's diameter of choice; the author's preference is 42 mm, then the entire area of the skin between the NAC and the Wise-pattern marking is de-epithelialized. Next, breast skin flaps with a thickness of 1 cm are raised superiorly toward the clavicle, degloving the breast parenchyma until the pectoralis fascia is reached. The dissection then proceeds in this plane until the clavicle is reached. Medial and lateral dermoglandular flaps are raised, respectively, off the medial and lateral portions of the pectoralis fascia. These flaps are pedicled on the chest wall, and the dissection need only proceed as far as necessary for mobilization of each flap superiorly to abut the central pedicle. In doing so, perforators are preserved at the base of each pedicle to supply the respective flaps. The lateral flap may be raised posterior to the posterior axillary line if needed; however, this increases the risk of fat necrosis. Centrally, the NAC is preserved on a pedicle of at least a 10-cm width. Once all flaps have been raised, the whole pocket is irrigated and hemostasis is verified.

After completing the dissection, the remainder of the procedure involves a tailored set of steps to reshape the breast based on aesthetic norms. The first portion involves suspending the newly raised pedicles to a permanent location on the chest wall. Starting with the central pedicle, the superior dermal edge of the keyhole pattern is tacked

to a rib periosteum along the previously marked breast meridian. The rib level is determined intraoperatively based on the position of the NAC in relation to the IMF after fixation, most often at the level of the second or third rib. Using the nondominant index and middle fingers to flank the rib in the intercostal space, a size braided permanent suture is used to take a bite through the pectoralis muscle and periosteum. The medial and lateral flaps are similarly secured to the periosteum of the same rib or one level lower, depending on the location that gives the desired breast shape. The point of fixation is chosen immediately medial and lateral to the meridian, respectively, to bring the superior parts of each flap adjacent to the central, akin to closing flower petals over a central pistil or stamen.

Additional fixation sutures are placed as needed to reinforce the suspension of the breast. Sutures are placed in a horizontal mattress fashion to invert the lateral flap dermis down onto the chest wall, using the pectoralis muscle as the anchor. These sutures can also be used to give the breast parenchyma a more natural, round shape and eliminate the bulging tissue in the axilla. Plication sutures are then placed to smooth the junction of the central flap with the medial and lateral flaps. A 2-0 absorbable suture is used, in an interrupted or running fashion, to bring the edges together and decrease the bulging tissue at the interface between the flaps. The final row of plication sutures is placed in the inferior pole of the breast to adjust the restore a more natural distance between the nipple and IMF. This maneuver also increases projection of the breast and corrects the pseudoptosis deformity. An intraoperative photograph of the result before skin closure is shown in **Fig. 2.**

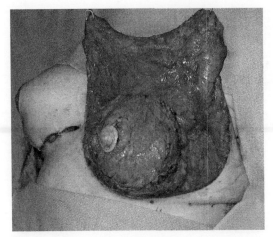

Fig. 2. Intraoperative photograph of the patient in **Fig. 3** showing the suspension of the medial, central, and lateral dermoglandular pedicles to the chest wall. Sutures have additionally been placed along the chest wall laterally to round the breast shape as well as plication sutures inferiorly to decrease the IMF distance. The dermis around the superior portion of the NAC has been released to drop the nipple position to a more natural location.

Finally, the breast skin flaps are redraped over the new breast contour. The NAC may need to be partially released if it sits at an inappropriate position on the chest wall. The NAC may be released partially by incising the dermis around it to allow inset into its keyhole. Once the result

is satisfactory, a drain is placed and closure is performed. Closure is performed with an absorbable suture, and cyanoacrylate glue is used to seal the incision. The breast is wrapped with an Ace bandage or other compression dressing.

Certain key points are worth mentioning:

- Constant redraping of the skin flap throughout the shaping process will guide adjustments to breast shape.
- To optimize symmetry, it is best to perform each step at the same time on both breasts rather than completing one breast then moving onto the other.
- Symmetry between sides is assessed frequently, and corrections are made at each sequential step before moving on to the next.

POSTOPERATIVE CARE

Patients should be seen on the first postoperative day to remove the dressings and check for any evidence of bleeding. If other procedures were performed concurrently, this may require staying overnight in the operative facility. Alternatively, they can be sent home and seen in the clinic the following day. The dressings are removed at that time, and an evaluation is made of symmetry and edema. Drains are assessed for quantity and quality of output. Once again, the breast is wrapped in compression dressing and patients are seen 5 to 7

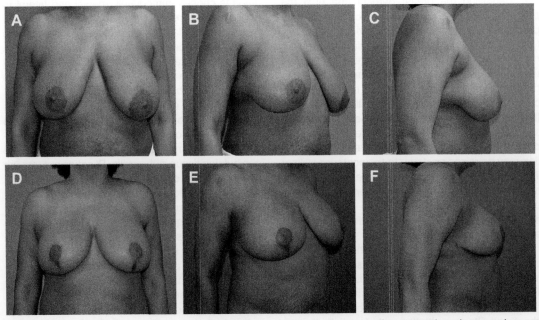

Fig. 3. A 55-year-old woman shown (*A–C*) preoperatively and (*D–F*) 18 months after DSPR. She subsequently went on to have autologous fat transfer to the breasts for enlargement (not shown).

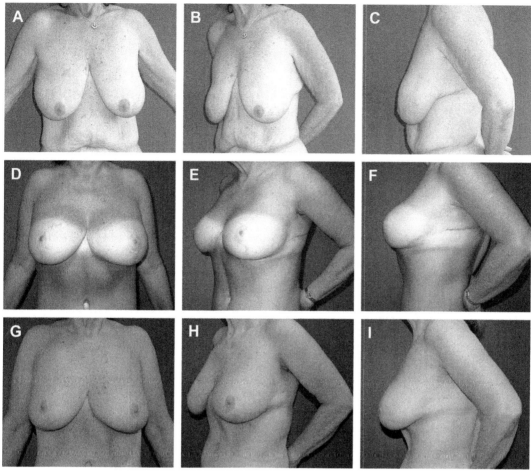

Fig. 4. A 53-year-old woman who lost 98 kg after laparoscopic gastric bypass presented to the author's office (A–C) almost 2 years after her bariatric surgery. She underwent DSPR, and her results are shown at (D–F) 1 year and (G–I) 10 years postoperatively. She had no revision surgeries, a notable example of the longevity of the procedure.

days later for a second visit. At that time, drains are usually removed per surgeon preference, typically if the output is less than 30 mL over a 24-hour period. Additionally, patients are transitioned into a brassiere without an underwire or a nonmedical compression garment of choice.

OUTCOMES

This technique has been used by the author for more than 15 years with predictable, lasting results. The most common complications noted are seroma and dehiscence, both minor problems that can generally be treated in the clinic.[8] Patients retain upper pole breast fullness many years postoperatively, likely because of the suspension of the dermis to the rib periosteum. **Figs. 3** and **4** demonstrate 2 different patients at short- and long-term follow-up.

SUMMARY

The technique of DSPRM is a useful procedure for patients with MWL with a typical presentation. The operation is tailored to the individual deformity, powerfully reshapes the breast, and can be safely combined with other commonly performed procedures. It is associated with minor complications that are easily treated in an office setting.

REFERENCES

1. Kahn S, Hoffman S, Simon BE. Correction of non-hypertrophic ptosis of the breasts. Plast Reconstr Surg 1968;41(3):244–7.
2. Regnault P. Breast ptosis. Definition and treatment. Clin Plast Surg 1976;3(2):193–203.
3. Coombs DM, Srivastava U, Amar D, et al. The challenges of augmentation mastopexy in the massive

weight loss patient: technical considerations. Plast Reconstr Surg 2017;139(5):1090–9.

4. Wong C, Vucovich M, Rohrich R. Mastopexy and reduction mammoplasty pedicles and skin resection patterns. Plast Reconstr Surg Glob Open 2014;2(8): e202–7.

5. Rubin JP. Mastopexy after massive weight loss: dermal suspension and total parenchymal reshaping. Aesthet Surg J 2006;26(2):214–22.

6. Losken A, Holtz DJ. Versatility of the superomedial pedicle in managing the massive weight loss breast: the rotation-advancement technique. Plast Reconstr Surg 2007;120(4):1060–8.

7. Oeffinger KC, Fontham ET, Etzioni R, et al. Breast cancer screening for women at average risk: 2015 guideline update from the American Cancer Society. JAMA 2015;314(15):1599–614.

8. Rubin JP, Gusenoff JA, Coon D. Dermal suspension and parenchymal reshaping mastopexy after massive weight loss: statistical analysis with concomitant procedures from a prospective registry. Plast Reconstr Surg 2009;123(3):782–9.

Bra-Line Back Lift

Joseph Hunstad, MD*, Charlie Chen, MD, Turkia Abbed, MD

KEYWORDS

- Bra-line back lift • Back contouring • Upper body lift • Back rolls

KEY POINTS

- Comprehensive upper back deformity, which includes laxity of the skin, excess adiposity, and redundant lateral breast tissue, can be corrected using the bra-line back lift.
- Candidates for the procedure have graspable soft tissue laxity in the mid and lateral upper backs. The resection pattern extends anteriorly to axillary line at the level of the inframammary fold.
- Preservation of loose areolar tissue over underlying muscle fascial will help minimize pain and swelling.
- The procedural learning curve is gentle for surgeons experienced in excisional body contouring with predictable results and satisfactory outcomes.

INTRODUCTION/OVERVIEW

The normal aging or fluctuations in weight has significant effects on the skin and fat appearance in the upper back.[1–23] Distribution of subcutaneous fat and differences in skin elasticity can create effects on the skin that are cosmetically and functionally unappealing to patients. These effects are further accentuated by natural zones of adherence for soft tissue in the body contour. Anatomic sequelae in the upper back in particular have been often overlooked. Natural upper torso adherence zones in the posterior midline create tether points that lead to both horizontal and vertical laxity.[1,4] A lampshade effect is created on the skin and soft tissue of the upper torso.[3] These tether points hinder contouring of the upper back from procedures such as lower body lifts by preventing transmission of forces to this area (**Fig. 1**). Contouring procedures of the lower and mid-trunk, in fact, may even accentuate these deformities in some instances.[4–10]

Treatment of this area must be tailored to the particular patient. Some may be candidates for standard tumescent liposuction or adjunctive liposuction procedures using laser or ultrasound.[1,4] Skin in the upper back is robust, with thicker epidermis and dermis to aid in retraction following liposuction. However, the thicker and more fibrous fat in the upper back may be more resistant to traditional methods of liposuction.[4] Because of this, many may be candidates for direct excision of this tissue.[1,4,24]

Excisional methods of excess tissue in the past have been described with skin resection in a dermatomal pattern. However, this tends to leave an oblique scar that is impossible to conceal in normal clothing.[1] These scars are often disfiguring. The authors present the bra-line back lift, a consistent and reliable method of addressing these issues by completely eliminating both excess skin and subcutaneous fat from the region while correcting excess skin laxity in both normal-weight and massive-weight-loss populations.

TREATMENT GOALS AND PLANNED OUTCOMES

The goals of the bra-line back lift are to consistently and safely eliminate the skin and subcutaneous fat from the posterior upper torso while correcting excess skin laxity. The well-accepted position of the scar beneath the bra line without the need for a drain enhances patient satisfaction

Disclosure Statement: The authors have nothing to disclose.
Hunstad Kortesis Bharti Cosmetic Surgery, 11208 Statesville Road, #300, Huntersville, NC 28078, USA
* Corresponding author.
E-mail address: Dr.H@HKCenters.com

Clin Plastic Surg 46 (2019) 77–84
https://doi.org/10.1016/j.cps.2018.08.010

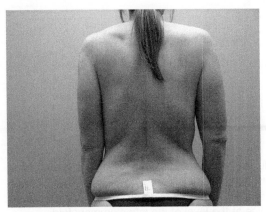

Fig. 1. Patients are evaluated for skin quality, stretch marks, subcutaneous adiposity, and excess or hanging skin. Note the tethering points that compromises a smooth transition of the upper back.

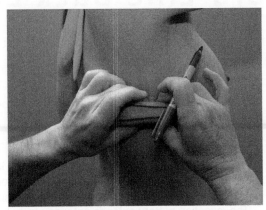

Fig. 2. Strong bimanual palpation helps to demonstrate the final outcome in terms of tissue resection. It shows the surgeon and patients the expected contour after resection.

and minimizes postoperative complications. Patients are able to achieve an ideal contour with relatively minimal morbidity and downtime. The procedure may be combined safely with other body-contouring procedures, such as reverse abdominoplasty, mastopexy, and breast reduction, to maximize patient outcomes.

PREOPERATIVE PLANNING AND PREPARATION

The patients are given a comprehensive understanding of body-contouring procedures and how they relate to their particular situation and deformity. Diagrams and photographs are reviewed and tailored to the patients' particular goals and desires. The authors discuss a comprehensive approach to the area of treatment and how it will affect their long-term goals.

Routine complete blood counts, comprehensive metabolic panels, and coagulation profiles are drawn and reviewed. Patients are instructed to discontinue any nonsteroidal anti-inflammatory drugs and herbal medications 2 weeks before surgery. Smoking is a relative contraindication.

PATIENT EVALUATION

Patients with concerns of upper back tissue excess are evaluated for skin quality, stretch marks, subcutaneous adiposity, and excess or hanging skin (see **Fig. 1**).

Most patients will grasp the redundant skin and excess adiposity of the upper back to demonstrate areas they would like to see improvement. In the full-length mirror, the surgeon shows the patients how much will be removed and the contour improvement that they will expect from the neck

to the back. Redundant tissue is firmly grasped with bimanual palpation to demonstrate the final outcome in terms of tissue resection (**Fig. 2**). The day of surgery, patients are encouraged to bring their most revealing bra or bathing suit top to plan the area of scar placement and ensure that their expectations will be met.

Patients are counseled on the importance of keeping the arms adducted until full tissue relaxation. Full range of motion will be permitted in 6 weeks or less.

PREOPERATIVE MARKINGS

Patients are marked in a standing position with arms at the sides. This position allows for the maximum amount of tissue to be safely removed. A standard photographic technique is used to record the entire lateral and upper back condition. These photographs consist of left and right lateral and oblique images as well as a posterior image with the patients' arms down at the sides.

The boundary of the patients' ideal scar position is marked to fall within the outlined margins of the bra or bathing suit top of choice (**Figs. 3** and **4**). If there is not a preferred undergarment, then the ideal final incision line is determined by first identifying the level of the inframammary fold bilaterally. This mark is transcribed across the back in a horizontal fashion.

Bimanual palpation is then used to strongly gather the redundant skin and excess adiposity such that it centers on the final incision line (**Figs. 5** and **6**). This technique is performed at multiple points across the ideal incision, and the line is marked superiorly and inferiorly. The markings are subsequently connected identifying the final area of resection. Because of the strong zone of

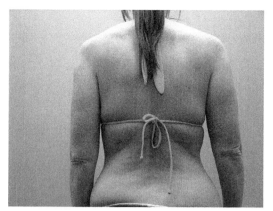

Fig. 3. Patients are encouraged to bring their most revealing bra or bathing suit top to plan the incision-line placement and ensure that their expectations will be met.

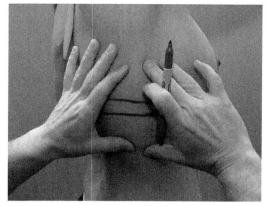

Fig. 5. Strong bimanual palpation is used to identify the resection pattern and center the superior and inferior resection markings on the final proposed incision line, marked in black.

adherence in the midline, the resection will be least at this position. The resection pattern is strongly tapered into the inframammary fold at the level of the anterior axillary line to avoid a dog-ear (**Figs. 7** and **8**). Realignment markings are made to aid in intraoperative assessment of resection patterns.

The marks are reviewed with patients with the aid of a mirror. A full set of postmarking photographs are also taken.

PATIENT POSITIONING

Following the induction of general anesthesia, patients are carefully turned to the prone position. Chest rolls are used along with padding at the knees and ankles. Sequential compression devices are used on the lower extremities.

Arms are placed on the adjustable arm boards with the elbows flexed and upper arms only

moderately abducted. This position aids in reducing tension on closure in the mid-axillary line. Adjustable arm boards allow further arm adduction, if needed, to decrease tissue tension during closure.

PROCEDURAL APPROACH

A penetrating towel clip is used to confirm preoperative markings and assess tension at multiple points (**Figs. 9–11**). Difficulty in closing the clamp signifies excessive tension and more conservative markings are adjusted accordingly. These markings are then subsequently tattooed with methylene blue at the realignment points (**Fig. 12**), which aids in reapproximation of tissues, as marked lines will invariably be wiped off during the procedure. These marks should be made

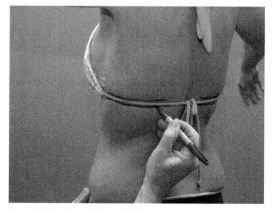

Fig. 4. The boundary of the patients' ideal incision position is marked to fall within the outlined margins of the bra or bathing suit top of choice.

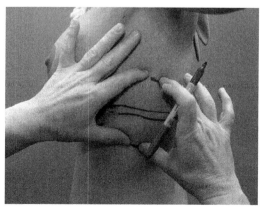

Fig. 6. This palpation is continued at multiple points to keep resection patterns within the areas of concealed tissue. Final closure line is marked in black.

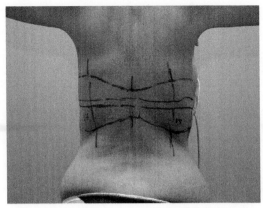

Fig. 7. Markings are connected to outline the superior and inferior resection patterns for the procedure. Because of the strong points of adherence, the narrowest area of resection will be in the midline.

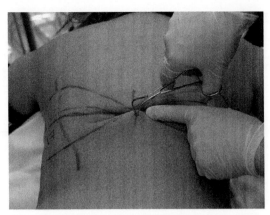

Fig. 9. Penetrating towel clamps are used to assess tension on incision lines at multiple points.

outside of the pattern of resection so that they may be seen at the time of closure.

Dilute lidocaine with epinephrine may be used to infiltrate the incision lines. In addition, the authors infuse the loose areolar tissue and incision lines above the muscular fascia with a dilute tumescent infiltration. Full prepping and draping is performed.

Incisions are made into the dermis. Electrocautery is then used to continue the incision through the dermis, sealing the subdermal plexus to minimize bleeding. Dissection proceeds, without beveling or undermining, straight down to the loose areolar plane above the muscle fascia. Leaving this layer of tissue will facilitate closure. It allows room for space-obliterating sutures.

The resection is completed and tissue passed off for weighing. Meticulous hemostasis is ensured. Skin edges are temporarily closed with

penetrating towel clamps, using previously placed realignment marks as reference points. A 3-layered closure is then performed to create space obliteration. This closure is done by taking bites of the superficial fascial system (SFS), then underlying muscular fascia, and then the opposite side of the superficial fascia (**Fig. 13**).

Taking accurate bites of the SFS layers is of vital importance to the closure. It is important to recognize that the SFS may seem to retract in relation to the overlying dermis when the towel clamps are placed. Understanding this and ensuring strong and accurate bites of this layer will optimize closure and decrease the chance of scar widening. Conveniently for the patients and surgeon, if this is performed meticulously, it eliminates the need for drains.

Based on tension, either a 0 or number 1 polyglactin (Vicryl; Ethicon Inc, Somerville, NJ) suture is used. The closure begins laterally and

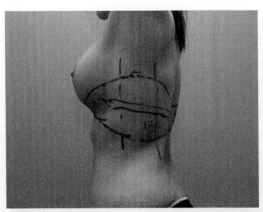

Fig. 8. As seen in this photograph, the widest margins of resection will fall within the area of the posterior axillary line, the most distant from the midline zone of adherence.

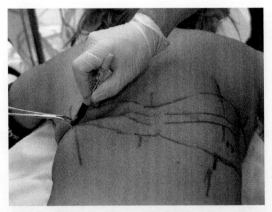

Fig. 10. Penetrating towel clamps are used to assess tension on incision lines at multiple points. Incision lines are reinforced or readjusted according to clamp tension.

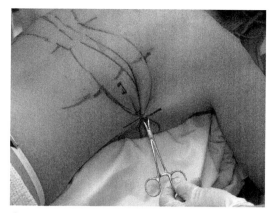

Fig. 11. Penetrating towel clamps are used to assess tension on incision lines at multiple points.

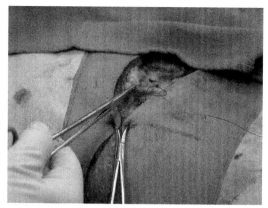

Fig. 13. Towel clamps are used to facilitate a temporary closure of the wound. A 3-point closure is performed by taking a bite of the SFS, then underlying muscular fascia, then the opposite side superficial fascia. Closure begins laterally and progresses medially.

progresses toward the spine, selectively removing towel clamps along the way. Towel clamps can be progressively used at selective points of higher-tension closure to ensure that good opposition is secured.

The deep dermis is closed with a 2 to 0 polyglactin (Vicryl) suture in a buried fashion. The final layer is finished with an intracuticular running 4 to 0 poliglecaprone suture (Monocryl, Ethicon Inc). The entirety of procedure may be performed with the patient in the prone position. Should this procedure be combined with a mastopexy, breast reduction, or reverse abdominoplasty, a temporary V-Y closure can be performed laterally as far as the table permits. Closure on the back can proceed and then the V-Y closure released when patients are subsequently turned supine.

The suture line is then treated with either tissue adhesive or taping. In taping, it is important to split

the tapes periodically to allow for swelling and to avoid shearing forces. This splitting avoids blistering and subsequent hyperpigmentation of the incision line.

POTENTIAL COMPLICATIONS AND MANAGEMENT

The most common complication after a bra-line back lift is scar widening. The primary author's experience reveals that patients have been unconcerned with the minor widening that may occur with the incision over time. Early experience with this method revealed widening concerning to patients to be the case in fewer than 5% of cases.[10] If this occurs, a scar revision is offered no sooner than 3 months after healing to allow for full relaxation of the tissues. These revisions subsequently do not widen.

Rarely, a patient may be concerned of a possible undercorrection. In these cases, additional resection can usually be performed under local anesthesia. Lateral dog-ears will generally

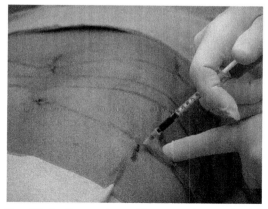

Fig. 12. Realignment markings are tattooed with methylene blue, as they will invariably be lost during the procedure. Note how the tattooing is performed outside of the resection pattern so that they may be seen at the time of closure.

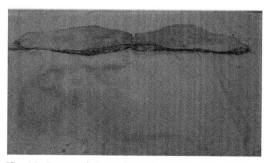

Fig. 14. Resected tissue from the bra-line back lift.

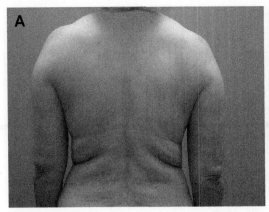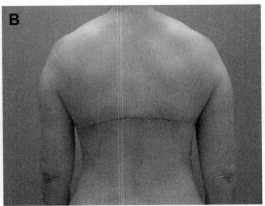

Fig. 15. (*A*) A 45-year-old woman who desired contouring to correct upper back skin and subcutaneous fat changes. (*B*) Early postoperative photograph at 2 weeks.

settle out over several months. Revision under local anesthesia is occasionally required.

Local wound-healing complications are managed with debridement and secondary intention healing or delayed primary closure. Seroma, hematoma, and infection have not been experienced in the authors' series; however, they are still discussed as a part of the informed-consent process. Should they occur, standard surgical techniques, including drainage, debridement, and wound care, are recommended.

POSTPROCEDURAL CARE

Patients are allowed to shower on postoperative day one. It is important to remind them to leave their arms adducted when shampooing their hair. Range of motion and arm abduction is increased gradually based on patient comfort. If abducting the arms is painful or creates undo tension, they are advised to scale back their activity. Common

sense in matters of activity is stressed with patients and their family. Skin tapes are changed weekly in clinic and removed after 4 postoperative weeks. Scar therapy is begun at that time, consisting of silicone cream application 3 times daily.

OUTCOMES AND EVIDENCE

Over a 17-year period, more than 77 procedures have been performed in the authors' practice either as isolated cases or in combination with others. The overall complication rate of scar widening requiring minor revision has been less than 5%. Even with minor widening, patients have been overwhelmingly pleased with the outcome and contour. There are no documented cases of infection, seroma, or hematoma over this period, which can be attributed to the 3-point space-obliterating closure that is used.

In postoperative photographs and patient records, this case series reveals increased patient

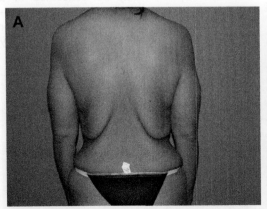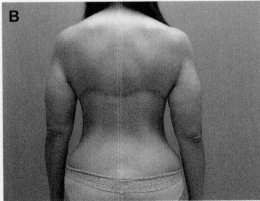

Fig. 16. (*A*) A 30-year-old woman with massive weight loss who desired contouring along upper back and flank. (*B*) Follow-up photograph at 3 months.

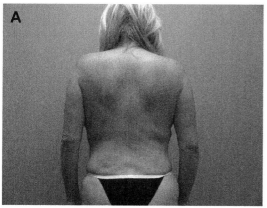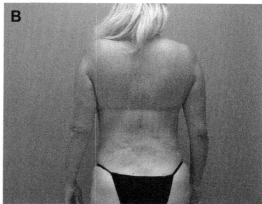

Fig. 17. (*A*) A 44-year-old woman who desired contouring to correct age-related changes along upper back and flank. (*B*) Follow-up photograph at 1 year.

satisfaction with minimal postoperative morbidity. The results were predictable and consistent throughout. See **Figs. 14–17** for some postoperative examples of resected tissue as well as patient examples.

SUMMARY

The transverse upper body lift that the authors refer to as the *bra-line back lift*[1,2,10] is a powerful tool that delivers consistent and safe results. It has proven useful for both normal-weight and massive-weight-loss patients who have experienced weight fluctuations and subsequent laxity. The procedure eliminates skin excess and adiposity from the upper back. The final scar is concealed beneath the bra line and tolerated well by patients. Complications are rare and can usually be managed by minor wound care or revision under local anesthetic. The overall patient satisfaction in the authors' practice has been universally high. Mastering this technique has a gentle learning curve and serves as a useful tool in the armamentarium of body contouring.

REFERENCES

1. Hunstad JP, Knotts CD. Transverse upper body lift. In: Rubin JP, editor. Body contouring and liposuction. Philadelphia (PA): Elsevier; 2013. p. 159–65.
2. Hunstad JP, Repta R. Bra-line back lift. Plast Reconstr Surg 2008;122(4):1225–8.
3. Solimen S, Aly A. Upper body lift. Clin Plast Surg 2008;35:107–14.
4. Shermak M. Management of back rolls. Aesthet Surg J 2008;28:348–56.
5. Strauch B, Rohde C, Patel MK, et al. Back contouring in massive weight loss patients. Plast Reconstr Surg 2007;120:1692.
6. Aly AS, Cram AE, Chao M, et al. Belt lipectomy for circumferential truncal excess: the University of Iowa experience. Plast Reconstr Surg 2003;111:398.
7. Van Geertruyden JP, Vandeweyer E, De Fontaine S, et al. Circumferential torsoplasty. Br J Plast Surg 1999;52:623.
8. Carwell GR, Horton CE. Circumferential torsoplasty. Ann Plast Surg 1997;38:213.
9. Hurwitz DJ. Optimizing body contour in massive weight loss patients: the modified vertical abdominoplasty. Plast Reconstr Surg 2004;114:1917–23 [discussion: 1924–6].
10. Hunstad JP, Urbaniak RM. Bra-line back lift. In: Strauch B, Herman CK, editors. Encyclopedia of body sculpting after massive weight loss. New York: Thieme; 2011. p. 230–9.
11. Shermak M. Body contouring. Plast Reconstr Surg 2012;129:963e.
12. Huemer GM. Upper body reshaping for the woman with massive weight loss: an algorithmic approach. Aesthetic Plast Surg 2010;34(5):561–9.
13. Strauch B, Herman C, Rohde C, et al. Mid-body contouring in the post bariatric surgery patient. Plast Reconstr Surg 2006;117(7):2200–11.
14. Gusenoff JA, Rubin JP. Plastic surgery after weight loss: current concepts in massive weight loss surgery. Aesthet Surg J 2008;28(4):452–5.
15. Aly AS. Upper body lift. In: Als AS, editor. Body contouring after massive weight loss. St Louis (MO): Quality Medical Publishing Inc; 2006. p. 235–60.
16. Rubin JP, Aly AS, Eaves FF III. Approaches to upper body rolls. In: Rubin JP, Matarasso A, editors. Aesthetic surgery after massive weight loss. Philadelphia: Elsevier; 2007. p. 101–12.
17. Cannistra C, Rodrigo V, Marmuse JP. Torsoplasty after important weight loss. Aesthetic Plast Surg 2006;30:667.
18. Gonzalez-Ulloa M. Belt lipectomy. Br J Plast Surg 1961;13:179.

19. Hamra ST. Circumferential body lift. Aesthet Surg J 1999;19:244.
20. Hunstad JP. Addressing difficult areas in body contouring with emphasis on combined tumescent and syringe techniques. Clin Plast Surg 1996;23:57.
21. Hunstad JP. Body contouring in the obese patient. Clin Plast Surg 1996;23:647.
22. Baroudi R. Flankplasty: a specific treatment to improve body contouring. Ann Plast Surg 1991;27:404.
23. Hurwitz DJ. Single stage total body lift after massive weight loss. Ann Plast Surg 2004;52:435.
24. Chamosa M. Lipectomy of fat rolls. Aesthetic Plast Surg 2006;30:417–21.

Arm Contouring in the Massive-Weight-Loss Patient

Paige L. Myers, MD, Ronald P. Bossert, MD*

KEYWORDS

- Brachioplasty • Arm contouring • Massive weight loss

KEY POINTS

- Brachioplasty for improved arm contour is a common procedure performed for the massive-weight-loss patient.
- There are several unique challenges to successful arm contouring in this population, such as redundant skin and loosening of fascial layers.
- Complications of brachioplasty are well documented and include seroma, dehiscence, nerve injury, and poor scar formation.
- Brachioplasty can be combined with liposuction as a safe and effective method for arm contouring without a higher risk of complications.

INTRODUCTION

Obesity continues to be a serious epidemic in North America and across the world with nearly one-third of Americans categorized as obese.[1] The benefits of bariatric surgery are well-documented[2–5] and as such, there is an appropriate increase in bariatric operations performed, with recent data reflecting nearly 200,000 performed annually.[6] The benefits of bariatric surgery include improvement in or resolution of type 2 diabetes mellitus, hypertension, hyperlipidemia, osteoarthritis, and obstructive sleep apnea.[7] Although patients' overall health is improved, new problems arise secondary to hanging redundant skin, such as intertriginous rashes, disabling pain, dermatitis, ulcerations, difficulty with hygiene, and limitation in activities of daily living.[3,8] Nearly 90% of patients undergoing bariatric surgery express a desire for body-contouring surgery to remove excess skin[1] for both cosmetic and functional reasons, including better physical quality of life and psychological well-being.[2–5]

The arms are a common area of redundant skin for which the massive-weight-loss population desires surgical improvement. The first brachioplasty procedure was described by Thorek[9] in 1930; although brachioplasty procedures have increased 235% since 2000 with more than 18,000 operations performed in 2017 alone.[10] Many iterations of the brachioplasty technique have been since developed to improve arm contour by removing redundant tissue and loose skin from the upper extremity and chest with different excisional patterns and addition of liposuction as adjunctive therapy. The ultimate goal of this procedure is to restore the ideal arm shape by removal with or without redistribution of soft tissues while minimizing scars and complications.[11]

RELEVANT ANATOMY

Hurwitz[11] eloquently describes the ideal female arm aesthetic shape as "tapering undulating cones extending from shoulders to elbow." In the

Disclosure: The authors have nothing to disclose.
Division of Plastic and Reconstructive Surgery, University of Rochester Medical Center, 601 Elmwood Avenue, Box 661, Rochester, NY 14642, USA
* Corresponding author.
E-mail address: Ronald_bossert@urmc.rochester.edu

Clin Plastic Surg 46 (2019) 85–90
https://doi.org/10.1016/j.cps.2018.08.011

youthful arm, skin is relatively tight with minimal adiposity. The toned musculature of the deltoid, biceps, and triceps constitute most of the external arm contour. The axilla is a shallow dome created by the tethered clavipectoral fasci and bordered by the triceps, latissimus dorsi, and pectoralis muscles.[11]

The complex fascial layers of the upper extremity and axilla are crucial to the overall contour of the arm. Just beneath the skin, the arm is shaped by 2 layers of adipose tissue separated by a superficial fascial system with variable integrity. The superficial, subdermal layer consists of vertically segmented adipose tissue and noteworthy neurovasculature. The deeper layer is a lamellar layer composed of horizontally oriented adiposity, which is the area more likely to store fat.[11–13]

Prone to injury, the medial antebrachial cutaneous nerves and medial brachial cutaneous nerves are located just beneath the superficial surface of the distal deep fascia layer. Anterior and posterior branches of the medial antebrachial cutaneous nerve originate at the level of the medial epicondyle. The main branch travels deep to the superficial fascial layer, running with the basilic vein in the distal one-third of the upper arm. It pierces the deep fascia 8 cm from the medial epicondyle. The medial brachial cutaneous nerve travels posterior the basilic vein with terminal branches 2 to 3 cm proximal to the medial epicondyle. Accompanying the sensory nerves, the basilic and cephalic veins, as well as the lymphatics, are located in the deep tissue layer of the arm, although the lymphatic basins are located more superficially in the axillary antecubital regions.[13,14]

DEFORMITY IN MASSIVE WEIGHT LOSS

There may be wide variability in the presentation of upper arm deformities exhibited by massive-weight-loss patients. Some may have minor ptosis with more residual lipodystrophy, whereas others may have developed major ptosis of the skin with minimal excess adiposity.[12,15,16] Regardless, the most common location for redundant skin in the massive-weight-loss patient is the posterior axillary fold and its extension down onto the lateral chest wall.[15] This causes flattening and obscures the otherwise aesthetic contour of the triceps.[11] Whereas the skin in the youthful arm is tight, hugging closely the underlying muscle and facial structures, the skin in the massive-weight-loss patient tends to be thin and lax (**Fig. 1**). Additionally, the axillary and clavipectoral fascia of the arm attenuates with age and weight changes, contributing to the arm resembling a "loose hammock."[17] This essentially deepens the axilla to give the deformity

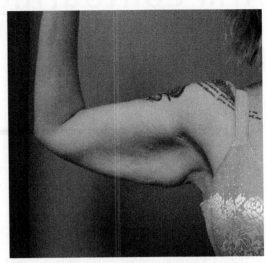

Fig. 1. The effects of weight loss on the contour of the arm, including attenuation of the skin and ptosis of the axilla.

of the hyperaxilla.[18] To worsen the problem, there is fullness in the lateral chest, generally from excess skin, which gives rise to a lateral bra roll. This causes the definition between the lateral borders of the pectoralis major and latissimus dorsi muscles to be blunted and a less aesthetically pleasing chest wall contour.[11,18]

Hurwitz and Jerrod[18] described the L-brachioplasty technique to specifically address the severe arm deformity in the massive-weight-loss patient. It is named as such due to the L-shaped excision extending from the elbow to axilla and down onto the chest wall. Extending the brachioplasty resection in this fashion helps tremendously to improve the contour of the axilla and the lateral chest wall.

Additional challenges in the massive-weight-loss patient include nutritional deficiency, changes in elastic and collagen fibers, and overall metabolic differences.[1] Because of these differences, there is nearly a twofold increase in complications for body contouring in massive-weight-loss surgeries compared with similar aesthetic procedures in the normal-weight population.[19]

TECHNIQUE

There are numerous approaches to brachioplasty in the massive-weight-loss population. The authors prefer to use the segmental resection approach, which has been well-delineated by Rubin and colleagues.[20] With the patient's elbow and shoulder at 90 degrees, begin by marking the bicipital groove. Next, a superior anchor line of incision is drawn with the skin on downward tension to simulate skin excursion. Keeping the skin under stretch is important to simulate the tension when closed for aggressive but appropriate resection. The proximal extent of the marked line is set high in the axillary dome and must extend inferiorly at a 90-degree angle onto the lateral chest wall. The inferior margin of resection is subsequently estimated by the pinch test and marked. Care must be taken to ensure the point of axillary resuspension does not impinge shoulder function (**Fig. 2**).

When in the operating room, the upper arm is prepared in the usual sterile fashion from lateral chest wall to the medial shoulder and distally to the level of the elbow. A sterile towel is wrapped around the arm just distal to the elbow to allow for maximal intraoperative manipulation (**Fig. 3**).

If liposuction is required, we recommend performing this before excision. It is important to note that concomitant liposuction is not to be performed in the region that is to be excised. This technique is rather used to more dramatically shape the posterior arm tissues that are otherwise not specifically addressed in traditional brachioplasty. To begin instilling tumescence into the subcutaneous fat of the posterior arm, a small incision is made at the elbow, cautiously avoiding the ulnar nerve.

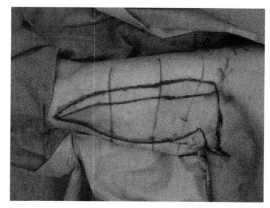

Fig. 3. Standard brachioplasty markings as outlined by Gusenoff and colleagues along with intraoperative draping.

Immediately after instilling tumescent solution, suction-assisted lipectomy is undertaken with 3-mm or 4-mm blunt-tipped cannula through the single port site at the elbow. This must be done expeditiously following infiltration to help avoid excess arm swelling and difficulties with closure following excision. Liposuction is then performed in radial fashion until the tissues of the posterior arm are uniform thickness and desirable contour.

Once the suction-assisted lipectomy portion is completed, the superior anchor line is sharply incised along with the anterolateral chest wall extension. A skin and subcutaneous fat flap is elevated as the dissection continues inferiorly. Meticulous care is taken to create a dissection plane superficial to underlying sensory nerves, as the medial antebrachial cutaneous nerve is located near the basilic vein in the distal upper arm (**Fig. 4**).

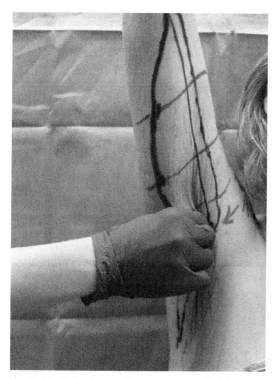

Fig. 2. Pinch testing in the preoperative holding area confirms the margin of resection, specifically at the point of the axillary resuspension, does not impinge shoulder function.

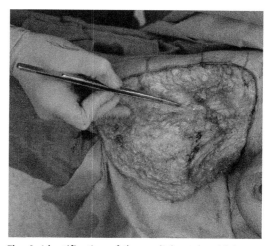

Fig. 4. Identification of the medial antebrachial cutaneous nerve along with the basilic vein under a thin layer of adipose tissue.

Tissues of upper arm are redraped to ensure there is no tethering before the margins of resection are reestimated. Heavy forceps are then used to transpose the superior anchor line under the dissected flap to once again estimate the appropriate margin of resection. The resection specimen flap is finally incised and segmentally resected to avoid overresection (**Fig. 5**). The superficial fascial layer of the flap at the point corresponding to the axillary dome is resuspended to the clavipectoral fascia using permanent 0 braided nylon sutures. Finally, the wound edges are temporarily reapproximated with staples before closure in layers over closed-suction drain and the arms wrapped in ace wraps from fingers to the axilla (**Fig. 6**).

COMPLICATIONS

Traditionally, common criticisms of brachioplasty include poor aesthetic quality due to scarring and relatively high complication rates. Complications are well documented and include seroma, dehiscence, nerve injury, lymphedema/lymphocele, and poor scar formation. Several modifications have been developed to minimize these complications and provide improved aesthetic results. To optimize scar placement, the final location will be in the bicipital groove. Thorough postoperative counseling regarding scarring is imperative to proper results. Seromas are prevented through the use of closed-suction drains and compression garments.

There are well-described strategies to decrease the risk of sensory nerve injury. Some investigators suggest that performing adjunctive liposuction within the excision margin minimizes dissection undermining. Additionally, it is advised to leave at least 1 cm of fat on the deep brachial fascia to prevent nerve damage. Astute knowledge of neurovascular anatomy is imperative to limit depth of

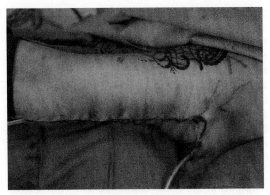

Fig. 6. The arm is stapled together before closure in layers over a closed-suction drain.

dissection and avoid injuring these critical structures.[11,13]

Surgical disruption of the lymphatic drainage in the upper extremity and axilla place patients undergoing brachioplasty at high risk for seromas or lymphocele formation with subsequent wound-healing problems. Knowledge of the locations of the lymphatics of the arm assists in protection against the risk of lymphatic drainage issues.[21–23] Many surgeons apply liposuction to their brachioplasty technique to assist in atraumatic dissection of tissue planes to avoid injury to lymphatics. Additionally, we recommend maintaining a relatively superficial plane in the distal arm and proximal axilla to avoid injury to important lymphatic basins located in these regions.

OUTCOMES

Gusenoff and colleagues[20] reported 100 patients prospectively in their experience with brachioplasty in the massive-weight-loss population, specifically analyzing complications when brachioplasty was combined with other excisional procedures. Ninety-six percent of all brachioplasty procedures performed were done so with concomitant body-contouring procedures on other anatomic regions. Twenty-four percent of patients underwent liposuction as well. Overall, their complication rate was 40.4%, with most being seromas. Longer operative time (>8 hours) was associated with increased overall surgical complications, including dehiscence, infection, and hematoma. Arm liposuction tended to increase arm-related complications in this study, although a follow-up study with a larger population by Bossert and colleagues[24] proved combining liposuction with brachioplasty is safe without an increased risk of complications. In this series, 144 massive-weight-loss patients undergoing brachioplasty with or without liposuction were prospectively followed with comparison of their

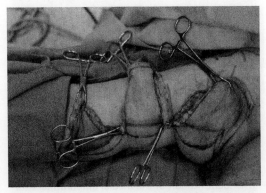

Fig. 5. Segmental resection is undertaken, allowing for safe surgical excision margins.

complication profile. The overall complication rate was 46%, with no statistically significant difference between patients who underwent excision with liposuction or with excision alone. The most common complication in this series was seroma for both excision and excision with liposuction, 23.1% and 19.1%, respectively. A similar study by de Runz and colleagues[25] compared brachioplasty alone with brachioplasty combined with other procedures. In this series, 36 patients underwent liposuction-assisted brachioplasty with a comparably low functional complication rate.

A large series by Knoetgen and Moran[26] looked at patients undergoing brachioplasty using an anterior incision. In their cohort, 76% were massive-weight-loss patients with an overall complication rate of 25%. An overwhelming majority (95%) of these complications were minor and included scarring, seroma, wound dehiscence, and nerve injury. The surgical revision rate was 12.5%.

Zomerlei and colleagues[19] retrospectively analyzed 96 patients who underwent brachioplasty. Fifty-three percent of these patients underwent concomitant surgeries and 53% underwent liposuction. Minor complications were common at 44.8% of the time and included infection and hypertrophic scarring. Major complications occurred 17.7% of the time, and minor complications occurred 44.8% of the time. Common complications included hypertrophic scar and infection with a 23.0% surgical revision rate, primarily for scar revision and improved contour. In accordance with Bossert and colleagues,[24] concomitant liposuction and/or other procedures were not associated with a significant increase in complications.

In a series of 31 patients, Symbas and Losken[27] described their outcomes of brachioplasty procedures. The overall complication rate was relatively low at 22% with a 16% surgical revision rate for dog-ears, contracture, scar malposition, and inadequate excision. Importantly, they found 94% of patients were satisfied with their results with improved self-esteem.

SUMMARY

Skin laxity of the arms is a common region of dissatisfaction in the massive-weight-loss population. Brachioplasty is an increasingly popular procedure performed for improved arm contour. There are several unique deformities presented in this population that must be addressed, such as redundant skin, posterior arm lipodystrophy, and loosening of fascial layers of the upper arm and chest wall. Common complications of brachioplasty include seroma, dehiscence, nerve injury,

and poor scar formation, but can be minimized with meticulous technique and knowledge of surgical anatomy. There are a number of well-described techniques to address skin laxity of the arms with similar, acceptable risk profiles. Additionally, brachioplasty can be combined with liposuction of the posterior arm as a safe and effective method for arm contouring without a higher risk of complications.

REFERENCES

1. Constantine RS, Davis KE, Kenkel JM. The effect of massive weight loss status, amount of weight loss, and method of weight loss on body contouring outcomes. Aesthet Surg J 2014;34(4):578–83.
2. Steffen KJ, Sarwer DB, Thompson JK, et al. Predictors of satisfaction with excess skin and desire for body contouring after bariatric surgery. Surg Obes Relat Dis 2012;8(1):92–7.
3. Manahan MA, Shermak MA. Massive panniculectomy after massive weight loss. Plast Reconstr Surg 2006;117:2191.
4. Singh KA, Losken A. The use of validated body image indices following panniculectomy. Ann Plast Surg 2011;66(5):537–9.
5. Warner JP, Stacey DH, Sillah NM, et al. National bariatric surgery and massive weight loss body contouring survey. Plast Reconstr Surg 2009;124:926.
6. The American Society for Metabolic and Bariatric Surgery. Estimate of bariatric surgery numbers, 2011-2015. Available at: https://asmbs.org/resources/estimate-of-bariatric-surgery-numbers on 11/22/2017. Accessed July 2, 2016.
7. Gurunluoglu R. Insurance coverage criteria for panniculectomy and redundant skin surgery after bariatric surgery: why and when to discuss. Obes Surg 2009;19:517–20.
8. Borud LJ, Warren AG. Body contouring in the post bariatric surgery patient. J Am Coll Surg 2005;203: 82–93.
9. Thorek M. Esthetic surgery of the pendulous breast, abdomen and arms in the female. Ill Med J 1930;58:48.
10. 2017 Plastic Surgery Statistics. American Society of Plastic Surgeons. Available at: https://www.plasticsurgery.org/documents/News/Statistics/2017/plastic-surgery-statistics-report-2017.pdf. Accessed March 1, 2018.
11. Hurwitz D. Brachioplasty. Clin Plast Surg 2014;41: 745.
12. Aly A, Cram AE, Pace D. Brachioplasty in the patient with massive weight loss. Aesthet Surg J 2006;26: 76–84.
13. Shermak M. Aesthetic refinements in body contouring in the massive weight loss patient: part 2. Arms. Plast Reconstr Surg 2014;134(5):726e–35e.

14. Chowdhry S, Elston JB, Lefkowitz T, et al. Avoiding the medial brachial cutaneous nerve in brachioplasty: an anatomical study. Eplasty 2010;10:e16.

15. El Khatib HA. Classification of brachial ptosis: strategy for treatment. Plast Reconstr Surg 2007;119:1337.

16. Gusenoff JA, Messing S, O'Malley W, et al. Temporal and demographic factors influencing the desire for plastic surgery after gastric bypass surgery. Plast Reconstr Surg 2008;121:2120–6.

17. Lockwood T. Brachioplasty with superficial fascial system suspension. Plast Reconstr Surg 1995;96:912–20.

18. Hurwitz DJ, Jerrod K. L-brachioplasty: an adaptable technique for moderate to severe excess skin and fat of the arms. Aesthet Surg J 2010;30:620–9.

19. Zomerlei TA, Neaman KC, Armstrong SD, et al. Brachioplasty outcomes: a review of a multipractice cohort. Plast Reconstr Surg 2013;131:883–9.

20. Gusenoff JA, Coon D, Rubin JP. Brachioplasty and concomitant procedures after massive weight loss: a statistical analysis from a prospective registry. Plast Reconstr Surg 2008;122:595–603.

21. Pascal JF, Le Louarn C. Brachioplasty. Aesthetic Plast Surg 2005;29:423–9 [discussion: 430].

22. Hill S, Small KH, Pezeshk RA, et al. Liposuction-assisted short-scar brachioplasty: technical highlights. Plast Reconstr Surg 2016;138:447e.

23. Gentileschi S, Servillo M, Ferrandina G, et al. Lymphatic and sensory function of the upper limb after brachioplasty in post-bariatric massive weight loss patients. Aesthet Surg J 2017;37(9):1022–31.

24. Bossert RP, Dreifuss S, Coon D, et al. Liposuction of the arm concurrent with brachioplasty in the massive weight loss patient: is it safe? Plast Reconstr Surg 2013;131:357.

25. de Runz A, Colson T, Minetti C, et al. Liposuction-assisted medial brachioplasty after massive weight loss: an efficient procedure with a high functional benefit. Plast Reconstr Surg 2015;135:74e.

26. Knoetgen J III, Moran SL. Long-term outcomes and complications associated with brachioplasty: a retrospective review and cadaveric study. Plast Reconstr Surg 2006;117:2219–23.

27. Symbas JD, Losken A. An outcome analysis of brachioplasty techniques following massive weight loss. Ann Plast Surg 2010;64:588–91.

Vertical Medial Thigh Contouring

Joseph Michaels, MD[a,b],*

KEYWORDS

- Thigh lift • Medial thigh lift • Vertical thigh lift • Thighplasty • Body contouring • Plastic surgery
- Skin • Weight loss

KEY POINTS

- Medial thigh laxity in the significant weight loss patient has both vertical and horizontal components that require correction for optimal results.
- Vertical thigh laxity is preferably corrected first with a lower body lift or extended abdominoplasty, both including mons pubis correction.
- Medial thighplasty with a groin crease excision (vertical vector only) is inadequate to correct thigh laxity of the middle and lower one-third of the medial thigh.
- Optimal medial thigh correction predominately requires a horizontal vector of pull leaving a vertical incision. Any residual vertical skin excess is excised within the groin crease.
- Preoperative evaluation, patient education, and managing patient expectations are essential to optimizing outcomes with medial thighplasty.

INTRODUCTION

Medial thighplasty continues to be one of the more challenging procedures for plastic surgeons. There are several factors that contribute to this:

- Anatomic concerns
- Patient expectations
- Scar placement
- Complications

Although the thighs are considered a single anatomic unit, the thighs need to be separated into medial and lateral components. There is not one procedure that can completely correct both components because the vectors of pull are different. The lateral thighs are best corrected with a vertical vector, whereas the medial thighs are best corrected with a horizontal vector. Because there are 2 different vectors of laxity, patients will often need 2 different procedures to optimally tighten the thighs. A lower body lift (LBL), and to a lesser degree an extended abdominoplasty, will help improve this vertical vector. A vertical medial thigh lift will correct the horizontal vector. This article focuses on the medial thighs. Correction of the lateral thighs will be addressed in Jean-Francois Pascal's article, "Buttock Lifting: The Golden Rules," in this issue.

The significant weight loss patient frequently presents with multiple areas of concern that they want corrected following their weight loss. Excess skin of the thighs is a common complaint for these patients. Not only is there skin redundancy of the thigh tissue itself, but relaxation of areas adjacent to the thighs can further contribute to the loose skin seen in the thighs. Laxity of the abdominal skin, the mons pubis, and the buttocks can worsen the appearance of the thighs. Correction of these bordering areas will have a direct improvement on the overall contour of the thighs (**Fig. 1**).

Disclosure: The author has nothing to disclose.
[a] Private Practice, Michaels Aesthetic & Reconstructive Plastic Surgery, 11404 Old Georgetown Road, Suite 206, North Bethesda, MD 20852, USA; [b] Department of Plastic and Reconstructive Surgery, Johns Hopkins Medicine, 601 North Caroline Street, Baltimore, MD 21287, USA
* 11404 Old Georgetown Road, Suite 206, North Bethesda, MD 20852.
E-mail address: drmichaels@josephmichaelsmd.com

Clin Plastic Surg 46 (2019) 91–103
https://doi.org/10.1016/j.cps.2018.08.014

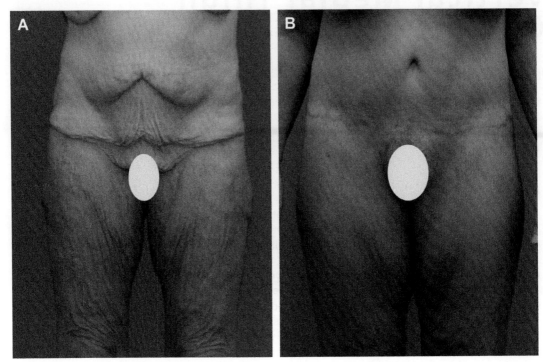

Fig. 1. (*A*) This 37-year-old woman, body mass index (BMI) of 26.8, lost 160 lbs. following bariatric surgery. She complained of skin laxity in her abdomen, inner and outer thighs, and buttocks. (*B*) She underwent a lower body lift (LBL) with mons pubis lift and buttock autoaugmentation. This case demonstrates how correction of adjacent structures to the thighs (abdomen, mons pubis, and buttocks) has a direct impact on thigh contour. The LBL will significantly improve the contour of the lateral and anterior thigh, but there is often only modest improvement of the medial thigh.

Patient expectations can be a challenge for medial thigh lift correction, because every patient wants short scars that are not visible. Patients will often stand in front of a mirror during their consultation and vertically lift all of their skin into their groin crease. Patients need to understand that this is not surgically possible. The groin crease is a fixed distance. The more skin that is removed vertically means the more skin mismatch there would be on the closure. This will also lead to more tension on this incision and adjacent structures such as the mons pubis. This can lead to a poor cosmetic result from skin bunching, widening of the scar, inferior scar migration, and labial spread. It is also not possible to correct the laxity in the middle and lower one-third of the thigh with just a groin incision. It requires a vertical incision with a horizontal vector of pull. Patients need to understand that a longer incision means more skin can be removed. If a patient does not want a vertical incision, they will have to accept that loose skin will remain in the middle and lower one-third of the inner thighs after their procedure. Proper counseling on scar placement and management of patient expectation are critical to having a successful patient outcome.

Of all the body contouring procedures, medial thigh lifts continue to have one of the highest complication rates among after weight loss body contouring procedures.[1–3] This is in part because of placement of the incisions in the groin crease. This region tends to naturally have higher bacterial counts than other areas of the skin due to higher moisture content. There is also tension on the incisions in the groin region, as well as shearing forces with ambulation and movements. All of these factors help contribute to higher complication rate seen with medial thighplasty, especially when the incision is limited to the groin crease.

Lewis originally introduced the thigh lift in 1957 where he described both a horizontal and vertical skin resection.[4] Lockwood later described a horizontal skin resection where the lower flap was anchored to Colles fascia to decrease tension and to minimize scar migration and widening.[5,6] Other investigators have also described techniques for a classical medial thigh lift that also uses a vertical vector of tension.[7–9]

Massive weight loss patients also commonly have medial thigh laxity and skin excess that can extend past the level of the knee and even onto the calf region. For this reason, a horizontal skin resection limited to the groin (vertical vector of pull) is often insufficient to correct the inner thigh deformity, because the forces of pull cannot adequately address the middle and distal thirds of the leg. A vertical medial thigh lift uses a longitudinal incision with a horizontal vector of pull to tighten the thigh like a cylinder. This allows adequate correction of the thigh laxity down the length of the leg and is the preferred method for treating the after weight loss patient.[1–3,10–13]

The laxity in the thigh has both a vertical and horizontal component. This vertical component is addressed by first correcting the abdomen, mons pubis, lateral thighs, and buttocks with LBL. An extended abdominoplasty will elevate the abdomen and mons pubis and correct some of the vertical vector but less so when compared with an LBL. Once the patient has fully recovered, the horizontal thigh laxity is addressed with a vertical media thigh lift. It takes at least 3 months between these staged procedures to allow swelling to return to normal and to make sure that the patient is once again medically and nutritionally optimized.

PATIENT SELECTION

After weight loss patients are unique in that they often have multiple anatomic areas of concern that they desire corrected. They also may have residual obesity-related medical issues and/or issues related to their weight loss surgery. A complete history and physical examination should be performed on all patients. Specific questions should be asked regarding their weight loss history, current body mass index (BMI), residual medical issues, their nutritional status, medications, social history, and any prior surgical procedures.

For the patient who presents with laxity limited to only the upper one-third of the medial thigh, a classical medial thigh lift can be performed. Most after weight loss patients have laxity that extends into the middle and distal one-third of the leg. For these patients, a vertical skin excision (horizontal vector) is the preferred method for correction (Figs. 2–5). The resultant scar will extend to just beyond where the laxity ends. In most cases, this will be just beyond the level of the knee.

Physical examination should focus on the degree of medial thigh laxity (Fig. 6), as well as an evaluation of adjacent areas that may be contributing to this laxity. These areas include the abdomen, lateral thighs, and the mons pubis. Assessment of the lower extremities for signs of lymphedema or peripheral vascular disease also needs to be documented.

Patients will often benefit from a tummy tuck or lower body lift before medial thigh contouring. This will first address the vertical vectors of laxity that are contributing to medial thigh laxity. During the consultation, it can be helpful to demonstrate the effects of an extended tummy tuck or LBL to patients. Lifting up on the lower abdomen will mimic an extended tummy tuck, whereas simultaneously lifting on the outer thighs will simulate a lower body lift. It is preferred to perform these procedures first and reserve medial thigh contouring for a second stage, but it is not uncommon to combine abdominoplasty and medial thighplasty when these are the patient's top 2 areas of concern.[14]

After weight loss patients will gain and lose their weight differently. A small subset of patients carries significant residual adiposity circumferentially in their thighs despite being at their goal weight. For patients who have circumferential thigh, a 2-stage approach will be considered. The first stage will be abdominoplasty or lower body lift combined with circumferential, debulking liposuction of the thighs. This allows for significant fat reduction from the thighs that will decrease the overall girth of the thighs. After waiting a minimum of 3 months for recovery and swelling to resolve, a vertical medial thigh lift can then be performed to remove the loose skin. This two-staged approach allows for the thighs to be made smaller than if done as a single stage. The downsides of this approach are 2 recoveries, increased cost, and a period of time in which the thighs look worse as a result of the deflated loose skin.

VERTICAL MEDIAL THIGHPLASTY
Patient Marking

Patients are marked in both the standing and frog-leg position. Standard photographs should be taken before marking the patient. These include anterior and posterior views of the thighs with legs in neutral position. Additional views are taken with each leg in abduction.

The patient is first marked in the standing position. A vertical line is drawn on the medial aspect of the thigh that cannot be seen from the front or back (Fig. 7). This line begins at the groin crease, posterior to the adductor muscle, and extends down the inner thigh ending in a curvilinear fashion and ends most commonly just below the knee. If the skin laxity ends in the middle one-third of the leg, a shorter vertical scar can be drawn. Although not common, the incision can also be extended onto the calf. This line represents the desired location of the final incision.

The patient is then asked to lie down on a stretcher in the frog-leg position. A skin

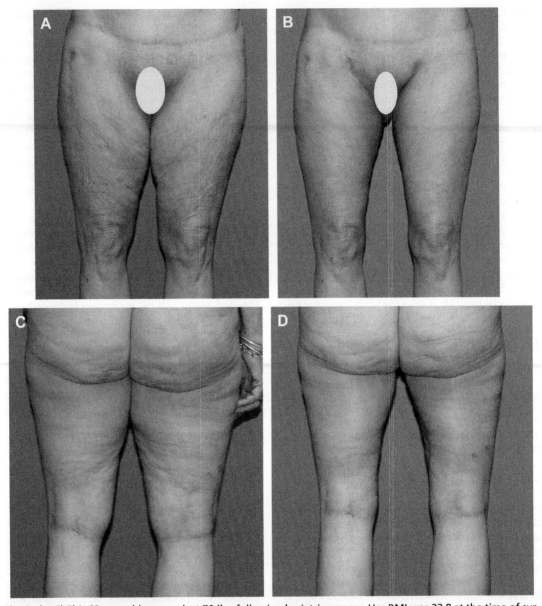

Fig. 2. (*A, B*) This 68-year-old woman lost 70 lbs. following bariatric surgery. Her BMI was 23.8 at the time of surgery. The patient had undergone previous extended abdominoplasty. (*C, D*) Postoperative views 9 months following vertical medial thigh lift.

displacement technique is then used to determine the anterior and posterior resection (**Fig. 8**A–F). This technique is performed at multiple points along the initial vertical marking. The markings are then connected and represent the anterior and posterior extent of the thighplasty excision. This resection pattern allows the leg to be closed as a cylinder with a horizontal vector of pull and a resultant vertical scar. Horizontal hash marks are also placed in several places to help guide closure.

There is often skin redundancy that remains at the anterior, superior aspect of the thigh. This redundancy lies parallel to the groin crease and is removed as a dog ear (**Fig. 8**G). Because this skin is just redundant, minimal vertical tension is placed on the groin crease incision. This minimizes the risk of scar widening and scar migration. Any areas of residual adiposity that fall outside of these lines are also marked for liposuction. The final markings are shown in **Fig. 8**H.

Patient Positioning and Preparation

The patient is brought into a prewarmed operating room to minimize the risk of

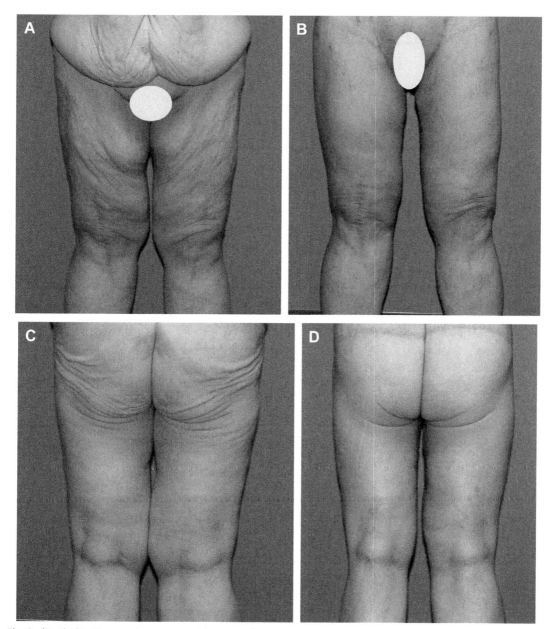

Fig. 3. (*A, B*) This 58-year-old woman, with a BMI of 28.3, lost 150 lbs. following bariatric surgery. She underwent previous panniculectomy and circumferential lower body lift. (*C, D*) Postoperative views 11 months following vertical medial thigh lift.

hypothermia.[15,16] A warming blanket is used under the patient. The patient is placed in the supine position with all dependent areas adequately padded and sequential compression devices are placed on the feet. Following anesthesia induction, a sterile Foley catheter is inserted and intravenous antibiotics are given. The lower abdomen, groin region, and the thighs are circumferentially prepped to below the knee.

Operative Technique

To minimize the risk of excessive swelling, the resection is completed on one side and the skin is temporarily closed with staples before proceeding to the contralateral leg. The area of proposed resection and any additional areas of excess adiposity are infiltrated with tumescent solution (12.5 mL of 1% plain lidocaine and 1 mL of 1:1000 epinephrine per 1 l lactated Ringer

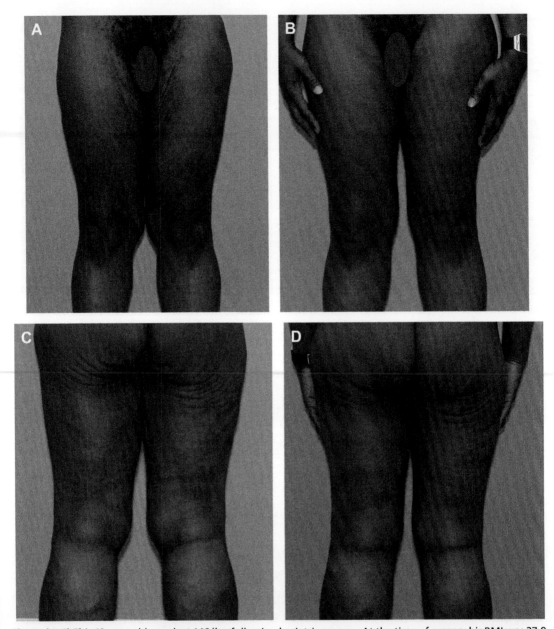

Fig. 4. (*A, B*) This 49-year-old man lost 146 lbs. following bariatric surgery. At the time of surgery his BMI was 27.9. The patient had undergone previous circumferential lower body lift and gynecomastia correction. (*C, D*) Postoperative views 11 months following vertical medial thigh lift.

solution). The volume of infiltrate should approximate the amount of estimated lipoaspirate. Excessive infiltration should be avoided because this can cause additional swelling in the postoperative period.

Liposuction is performed using power-assisted liposuction to debulk excess adiposity in the zone of resection and to allow for optimal skin removal (**Fig. 9**A). It also assists in skin removal by delineating the correct plane of dissection during resection. Additional areas of residual adiposity

are also liposuctioned to their desired contour. Liposuction is not performed in patients who have a low BMI or who have inner thighs that are significantly deflated.

Following liposuction, a pinch test is performed to confirm the area of resection (**Fig. 9**B). In some cases, additional skin can be removed following liposuction and this is marked as indicated. To minimize the risk of overresection and failure to close the incision, both the anterior and posterior incisions are not incised at the same time. The

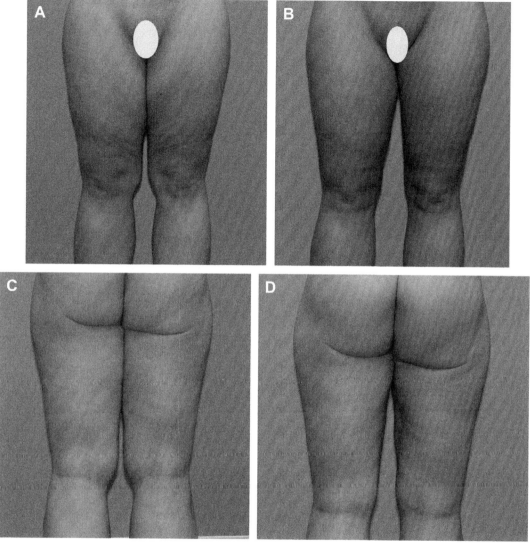

Fig. 5. (*A, B*) This 28-year-old woman, with a BMI of 29.0, lost 115 lbs. following bariatric surgery. She underwent previous circumferential lower body lift and mastopexy/augmentation. (*C, D*) Postoperative views 7 months following vertical medial thigh lift.

anterior vertical incision is made first and carried down through the superficial fascia to the residual adipose tissue overlying the deep fascia to the thigh musculature. The previously performed liposuction will result in a honeycomb appearance that helps with dissection and identification of the greater saphenous vein (**Fig. 9C**). An attempt should be made to maintain this structure in all cases, although this is not always possible. Dissection is carried out to the estimated posterior line of resection.

At this point, serial resections are performed to minimize the risk of excessive tension or overresection and failure to close the leg. This process is started distally and progresses proximally.

Following removal of each section, staples are used to temporarily approximate the skin and to help minimize swelling (**Fig. 10A–C**).

At the proximal aspect of the thigh, there is frequently a dog ear of skin at the superior aspect of the anterior thigh skin. This skin is marked with a pinch test and excised parallel to the groin crease (**Fig. 10D**). Minimal tension is used to estimate the skin excess. This technique avoids a triple point at the groin crease minimizing the risk of wound complications. Most of this skin lies anterior to the adductor tendon insertion. The plane of dissection becomes more superficial in this area due to concern for injury to the femoral lymphatic basin and the structures within the femoral triangle. In

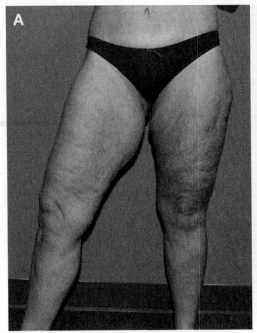
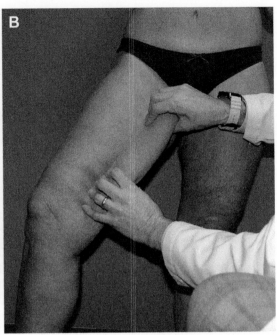

Fig. 6. (*A*) Laxity in the medial thigh can best be seen with the leg in abduction and the knee flexed. (*B*) By pinching the medial thigh skin with a horizontal vector of pull, the patient can see the effect of a vertical medial thigh lift.

this region the plane of dissection is just deep to the superficial fascial system (SFS).

If necessary, this dog ear extension can extend superiorly and connect to a previous abdominoplasty or LBL incision. If additional thigh tissue needs to be excised, the previous abdominoplasty

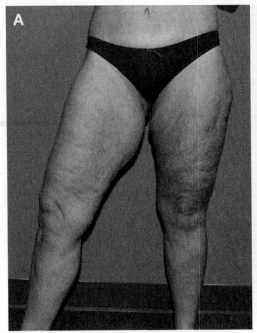

Fig. 7. In the standing position, the desired placement of the final incision line is marked on the medial aspect of the thigh so that it cannot be seen from the front or the back.

or LBL incision can be opened horizontally to facilitate the closure. The incision should never extend more superior than the patient's old incisions on the abdomen.

Once the resection has been completed and all incisions temporarily closed with staples, the same steps are performed on the contralateral thigh (**Fig. 11**A, B). Before formal closure, a #15F fluted Blake drain is placed and brought out proximally through a separate stab incision. The medial thigh skin usually has a very thin dermal layer and it may be challenging to get a 3-layer closure, so often a 2-layer closure needs to be performed. The vertical thigh incision is closed first. When the 2-layer closure is performed, the SFS and deep dermis are closed together with interrupted 0-Vicryl sutures. A running intracuticular 3-0 Monocryl stitch is then used to approximate the skin. If there is a good dermal layer, the SFS is first closed with a 0 Vicryl, followed by 3-0 Monocryl in both the deep dermis and intracuticular level. Where the vertical incision meets the horizontal groin excision, the closure is reinforced with 0-Vicryl sutures in the SFS that also incorporate Colles fascia in the cephalad tissue. The remainder of the closure posterior to the adductor tendon insertion is closed in a similar fashion to the vertical incision. Anterior to the adductor tendon, 3-0 Monocryl sutures are placed in the dermal and intracuticular layers (**Fig. 11**C).

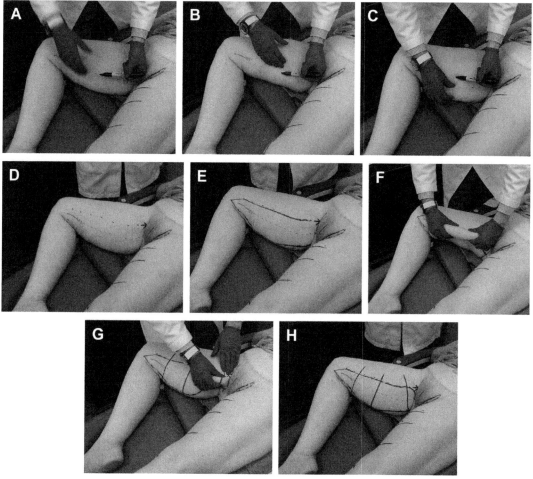

Fig. 8. (A–E) A displacement method is used, based on the desired scar position (*blue line*), to mark the anterior and posterior extent of the resection. (F) A pinch test is used to confirm closure without excessive tension. (G) The excess skin that remains at the anterior, superior aspect of the thigh is marked as a dog ear parallel to the groin crease. (H) Final thigh markings (the *arrow* represents the insertion of the adductor muscle tendon).

Marcaine 0.25% with 1:200,000 is injected into the incision line to help with postoperative comfort. Dermabond is used to seal the incision. Non-adherent dressings and loosely placed elastic wrap bandages are then placed.

Postoperative Care

When performed as a stand-alone procedure, the thighplasty is performed on an outpatient basis. When it is combined with additional procedures, patients frequently will be placed in observation

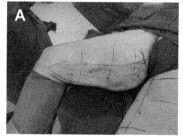
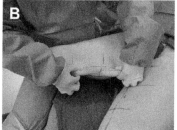
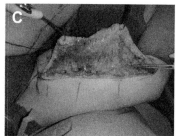

Fig. 9. (A) Debulking liposuction is performed in the estimated area of resection to help with dissection of the skin flap and to maximize the skin resection. (B) A pinch test is then used to confirm the anterior and posterior lines of resection. (C) Liposuction will facilitate flap dissection by making a honeycomb appearance during dissection. It also allows for easy identification of the saphenous vein (seen adjacent to pickup forceps).

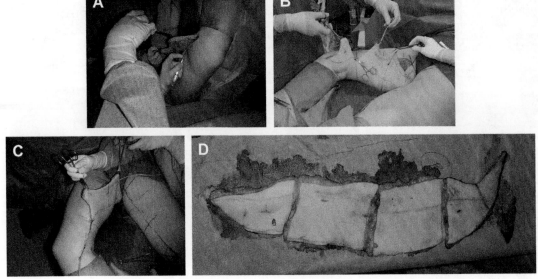

Fig. 10. (*A–C*) Serial resections are performed to minimize the risk of overresection and failure to close the incision. This is performed in a distal to proximal fashion. Each section is then temporarily closed with staples to minimize swelling before excision of the next area. (*D*) Serial excision specimens shown with the small dog ear of redundant tissue at the anterior, superior aspect that was excised parallel to the groin crease (*right* side of picture).

status and are discharged the day following surgery. To minimize the risks of venous thromboembolism, patients are instructed to ambulate the day of surgery. They are also started on low-molecular-weight heparin (LMWH) beginning 8 hours after surgery for 2 weeks.[17,18] Patients who have a hereditary coagulopathy or have other high-risk factors are given a preoperative dose of subcutaneous dose of unfractionated heparin (UH).[19] Although there is no increased incidence of bleeding

diathesis with preoperative heparin, the reversibility of UH is preferred as compared with LMWH.

To minimize tension on the incision, patients are instructed to shuffle step for the first few days and are advised not to abduct the legs more than 45°. The elastic wrap can be adjusted as necessary, because swelling has a tendency to peak at 48 to 72 hours and the dressing may feel too tight. Groin crease dressings are changed more frequently to help keep the incision dry. It is

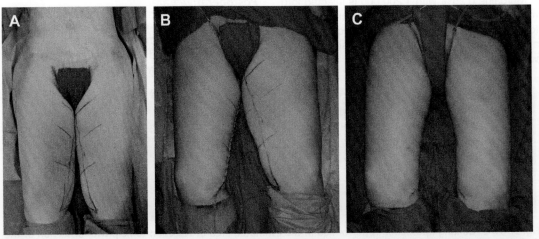

Fig. 11. (*A*) Preoperative pictures of the medial thighs. (*B*) Temporary closure of the right thigh following medial thigh skin resection compared with the contralateral thigh before resection. (*C*) Final closure of both medial thighs.

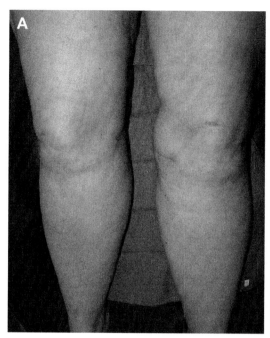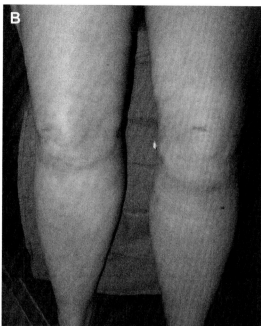

Fig. 12. (*A*) Postoperative left knee seroma. (*B*) This patient had return of her seroma following multiple aspirations. A stab incision was made in the media thigh scar into the seroma cavity and a wick left in place to allow the area to drain.

important to keep the groin area as dry as possible to prevent excessive moisture from building and to minimize the risk of wound healing complications. The patient is placed in a compression garment at their first postoperative visit and is asked to continue wearing it for 6 weeks. Care must be taken to make sure the garment does not disrupt the incision line, especially in the groin region.

Patients are kept on antibiotics until the drains are removed. The drains are removed when their output is less than 30 mL per day. This typically occurs 7 to 14 days following the procedure. Oral narcotic pain medications are used for patient comfort. Patients are seen in the office at 1 week, 4 weeks, 3 months, 6 months, and at 1 year.

Lower body exercises are allowed after 6 weeks, whereas upper body exercises can be started at 2 weeks. Scar treatments can be started at 2 to 3 weeks once the Dermabond adhesive falls off. Patients are told to minimize direct sunlight to the incisions and are instructed to use high-SPF sunscreen when the area is exposed. Patients are told the scar will continue to mature for up to 2 years.

Complications

When compared with other body contouring procedures, medial thighplasty has some of the highest complication rates. Recent published data showed complication rates ranging from 45% to 68%.[1–3] Most of these complications are minor and can be managed in the office on an outpatient basis. The most commonly observed complications are wound dehiscence (17%–51%), seroma (10%–25%), and infection (1%–15%).

Wound dehiscence often occurs 1 to 3 weeks after the procedure. It is most commonly managed with local wound care that may require some minor debridement in the office. These areas are generally less than several centimeters. Although attempts to reapproximate these areas can be made, they often fail due to the tension or shearing forces that caused them to occur in the first place. Wound care consists of cleaning the area daily and applying mupirocin 2% ointment and a dry dressing to the area daily. If the area is large enough to be packed with a wet to dry dressing, the patients are instructed to do this daily and then begin the antibiotic ointment once the area gets smaller. Silver nitrate may also need to be used in areas of hypergranulation tissue formation to allow for faster epithelialization of the wounds.

Seromas are the second most common complication seen with medial thighplasty. It can be seen within several weeks following drain removal and is most commonly seen around the knee region given dependent gravity and the rich lymphatic supply around the knee. Needle aspiration and compression is recommended twice weekly until it resolves. If the seroma persists, a small incision is made through the existing thigh incision and into the seroma cavity (**Fig. 12**). A wick is left in place for up to 3 days to allow the cavity to decompress. Then the patient is asked to place additional compression on the area. Patients are placed on antibiotics while the wick is in place. Excision of the seroma cavity may be necessary if more conservative interventions fail.

Infection rates have varied among recent published data. All patients are kept on oral antibiotics in the immediate postoperative course when the drains are in place. Generally a first-generation cephalosporin is used. Cellulitis around the incision line is the most commonly seen infection and can be managed with oral antibiotics. It is preferred to cover for both Streptococcus and Staphylococcus species and place patients most commonly on Cephalexin and Doxycycline. If there is drainage from the leg, a wound culture is performed and checked for sensitivities. In rare cases, admission for intravenous antibiotics is needed.

Although the incidence of venous thromboembolism in thigh lift patients is low, it is a reported risk. All patients are placed on postoperative LMWH for 2 weeks. If a patient is considered high risk, they will get a dose of preoperative UH and then postoperative LMWH for 4 weeks.

All patients should be counseled about the potential for prolonged swelling (up to 6 months) and about the possibility of chronic edema. Although the incidence has been very low, some reports show it can occur in up to 30% of patients.[20,21] Patients who have preexisting edema should be told that this might worsen after medial thighplasty and deferral of medial thighplasty should be considered on case-by-case basis.

SUMMARY

Body contouring after significant weight loss continues to be one of the fastest growing subsets within this field. Patients often complain of medial thigh laxity in addition to other areas they want corrected. Medial thighplasty can be a discouraging procedure for plastic surgeons to perform given its high complication rate. It is preferred to correct the vertical laxity component that contributes to medial thigh laxity by first performing a lower body lift or extended abdominoplasty. Residual medial thigh skin excess is usually due to a horizontal vector of laxity and is best corrected with a vertical medial thigh lift. Preoperative evaluation, patient education, and managing expectations are critical to optimize results. Although these procedures can be challenging for plastic surgeons, patient satisfaction for medial thighplasty can be very high.

REFERENCES

1. Gusenoff JA, Coon D, Nayar H, et al. Medial thigh lift in the massive weight loss population: outcomes and complications. Plast Reconstr Surg 2015;135:98–106.
2. Xie SM, Small K, Stark R, et al. Personal evolution in thighplasty techniques for patients following massive weight loss. Aesthet Surg J 2017;37: 1124–35.
3. Capella JF, Matarasso A. Management of the postbariatric medial thigh deformity. Plast Reconstr Surg 2016;137:1434–46.
4. Lewis JR Jr. The thigh lift. J Int Coll Surg 1957;27: 330–4.
5. Lockwood TE. Fascial anchoring technique in medial thigh lifts. Plast Reconstr Surg 1988;82:299–304.
6. Lockwood T. Lower body lift with superficial fascial system suspension. Plast Reconstr Surg 1993;92: 1112–22 [discussion: 1123–5].
7. Le Louarn C, Pascal JF. The concentric medial thigh lift. Aesthetic Plast Surg 2004;28:20–3.
8. Shermak MA, Mallalieu J, Chang D. Does thighplasty for upper thigh laxity after massive weight loss require a vertical incision? Aesthet Surg J 2009;29:513–22.
9. Spirito D. Medial thigh lift and DE.C.LI.VE. Aesthetic Plast Surg 1998;22:298–300.
10. Capella JF. The vertical medial thigh lift. Clin Plast Surg 2014;41:727–43.
11. Mathes DW, Kenkel JM. Current concepts in medial thighplasty. Clin Plast Surg 2008;35:151–63.
12. Hurwitz DJ. Medial thighplasty. Aesthet Surg J 2005; 25:180–91.
13. Cram A, Aly A. Thigh reduction in the massive weight loss patient. Clin Plast Surg 2008;35: 165–72.
14. Coon D, Michaels Jt, Gusenoff JA, et al. Multiple procedures and staging in the massive weight loss population. Plast Reconstr Surg 2010;125:691–8.
15. Coon D, Michaels J, Gusenoff JA, et al. Hypothermia and complications in postbariatric body contouring. Plast Reconstr Surg 2012;130:443–8.
16. Kenkel JM, Lipschitz AH, Luby M, et al. Hemodynamic physiology and thermoregulation in liposuction. Plast Reconstr Surg 2004;114:503–13 [discussion: 514–5].
17. Michaels J, Coon D, Mulvey CL, et al. Venous thromboembolism prophylaxis in the massive weight loss patient: relative risk of bleeding. Ann Plast Surg 2015;74:699–702.
18. Hatef DA, Kenkel JM, Nguyen MQ, et al. Thromboembolic risk assessment and the efficacy of enoxaparin prophylaxis in excisional body contouring surgery. Plast Reconstr Surg 2008;122:269–79.

19. Friedman T, O'Brien Coon D, Michaels VJ, et al. Hereditary coagulopathies: practical diagnosis and management for the plastic surgeon. Plast Reconstr Surg 2010;125:1544–52.

20. Moreno CH, Neto HJ, Junior AH, et al. Thighplasty after bariatric surgery: evaluation of lymphatic drainage in lower extremities. Obes Surg 2008;18: 1160–4.

21. Ellabban MG, Hart NB. Body contouring by combined abdominoplasty and medial vertical thigh reduction: experience of 14 cases. Br J Plast Surg 2004;57:222–7.

Face and Neck Lifting After Weight Loss

Joshua T. Waltzman, MD, MBA[a],*, James E. Zins, MD[b], Rafael A. Couto, MD[b]

KEYWORDS

- Facelift • SMAS • Platysmaplasty • Fat transfer • Massive weight loss

KEY POINTS

- The degree of facial aging after massive weight loss will be affected by age, amount of weight loss, rapidity of weight loss, and degree of loss of skin elasticity.
- Longer incisions along the posterior hairline are often necessary to remove excess skin low in the neck and to avoid hairline step-offs.
- Wide undermining of the face and neck is required to allow for mobilization of excess skin and access to the mobile superficial musculoaponeurotic system.
- Midface volumizing with selective placement of fat injections into the deep malar compartment is a useful adjunct technique in this patient population.

INTRODUCTION

Bariatric surgery has become increasingly common in the treatment of obesity and its comorbidities. Whether through surgical intervention or diet and exercise alone, massive weight loss (MWL) has a profound effect on reducing body fat and related disease[1]. However, it often results in skin redundancy that can be emotionally and psychologically distressing, and even physically cumbersome for the patient. Along with the rise in bariatric surgery, we have seen a rise in body-contouring procedures meant to address the excess skin and tissue laxity that results. Most of the weight that is lost comes from the trunk and extremities. It stands to reason, therefore, that MWL patients seek body-contouring procedures more frequently than facial procedures. However, there also can be profound changes in the face and neck, which can lead to the appearance of accelerated facial aging.

The degree of facial aging will be affected by the following[2,3]:

- Age
- Amount of weight loss
- Rapidity of weight loss
- Degree of loss of skin elasticity

In the face, skin redundancy typically tends to exceed superficial musculoaponeurotic system (SMAS) laxity. This may result in any or all of the following: an aged appearance with pronounced submalar hollows, deepened nasolabial folds, heavy jowling, marionette lines, and an obtuse cervicomental angle with central neck skin excess. In the upper third of the face, this can result in temporal hollowing and prominence of the lateral orbital rim. The midface and lower face/neck contain more subcutaneous fat, thus the effects of MWL are usually more apparent in this region. Although MWL patients are oftentimes able to conceal other areas of their body with shaping garments and clothing, the face and neck are areas that cannot be hidden. Although the literature is replete with body-contouring technique and outcome articles, there is a paucity of information on specifically

Disclosure Statement: The authors have nothing to disclose.
[a] Private Practice, Waltzman Plastic and Reconstructive Surgery, 3828 Schaufele Avenue, #360, Long Beach, CA 90808, USA; [b] Department of Plastic Surgery, Dermatology and Plastic Surgery Institute, Cleveland Clinic, 9500 Euclid Avenue, A60, Cleveland, OH 44195, USA
* Corresponding author.
E-mail address: drwaltzman@waltzmanplastics.com

Clin Plastic Surg 46 (2019) 105–114
https://doi.org/10.1016/j.cps.2018.08.012

addressing facial rejuvenation in this growing patient population.[2,4,5]

In general terms, the same concepts of face and neck lifting that apply to non-MWL patients hold true for the MWL population. However, there are several modifications that need to be considered for successful outcomes.

PREOPERATIVE MANAGEMENT

Analogous to other anatomic regions of the body after MWL, adequate time needs to be allowed for any residual skin contraction to take place. If facelift is performed while the patient is continuing to lose weight, there is a higher risk of recurrent laxity and volume deflation that can increase the chances of a suboptimal correction. Therefore, it is recommended that facelift surgery be deferred for a minimum of 6 months to 1 year after the patient's weight has stabilized.

Collaboration with the patient's primary care physician is recommended. A full metabolic workup to assess the possibility of malnutrition is important. Serum glucose should be measured and optimized before surgery. Although many MWL patients observe improved glucose control with weight loss, there can still be abnormalities that need to be addressed. It is also important to evaluate for anemia, electrolyte abnormalities, and vitamin deficiencies.[6] Routine electrocardiogram should be performed on all MWL patients to detect any cardiac arrhythmias or abnormalities.

As with most plastic surgery procedures, it is imperative to assess emotional stability and set proper expectations. Those patients with a marked skin excess should be counseled that a fully tightened neck and jawline may not be possible given the loss of skin elasticity. It is strongly advisable to counsel patients that revision procedures may be necessary to obtain optimal results.

A thorough facial analysis should be performed as part of the preoperative workup. Volume loss can occur in the temples, midface, buccal hollows, nasolabial groove region, and perioral area. Skin excess is commonly found along the jowls and submental region. Analysis of facial bone structure is helpful in assessing preoperative asymmetries. Common measurements include the bizygomatic distance, bigonial distance, and chin projection, as well as an analysis of facial height. Asymmetries or significant deviations from the norm noted preoperatively can be discussed with the patient. This allows time to set expectations, and decide what can realistically be achieved with surgery.

Preoperative photographs are a requisite to the complete preoperative management of the facelift patient. Photos should be obtained in front of a standardized background with reproducible lighting. Angles should include anterior, oblique, and lateral views. Care should be paid to the level of Frankfort horizontal.[7] Several degrees of deviation in tilt of the face can make a significant impact on the appearance of the neck and cervicomental angle. Consistent photography will allow for accurate comparison and evaluation of results.

OPERATIVE TECHNIQUE

Several investigators in the peer-reviewed literature have described their modified approach to the MWL facelift patient, and for the most part share many of the same ideas.[2,4,5,8] The sections that follow are a detailed description of these modifications. Any significant differences in approach between surgeons are specifically mentioned and referenced.

Facelifts for the MWL patient are performed under general anesthesia in an accredited outpatient surgery center or hospital facility. The patient should be marked in a seated upright position to visualize the full effect of gravity on the tissues. Useful landmarks include the extent of planned cheek dissection, location of the jowls, and any prominent platysmal bands that will need specific attention. The exact location of the incisions can be marked at this time, or in the operating room, as the position of the ear and hairline do not change significantly with position of the head.

Patients should receive a single dose of perioperative intravenous antibiotics. As of the writing of this article, 2 g of cefazolin (or equivalent) is the standard dosing, provided the patient does not have an allergy to cephalosporin antibiotics. Postoperative antibiotics are not administered, nor are there data to suggest their necessity. Sequential compression devices are applied to the lower extremities before the induction of anesthesia.[9] Once intubated, the endotracheal tube should be secured to the teeth with either a silk suture or 26-gauge wire to prevent tube migration. Securing the tube in this manner allows easy manipulation of the head and tubing during the surgery and provides unobscured views during the submental neck dissection. The patient is then prepped down to the level of the clavicles and draped in the usual sterile fashion. Any planned fat grafting donor sites are also prepped and squared off with towels at this time as well.

Incision Placement

One of the major differences in performing a facelift in the MWL patient is the length and position of the preauricular and postauricular incisions.

Longer incisions along the posterior hairline are necessary to remove excess skin low in the neck and to avoid hairline step-offs. For the preauricular incision, the anterior hairline incision may be preferable for the same reasoning. The large amount of skin excess and redundancy in the neck needs to be accommodated in a horizontal vector, which is best removed with an extended posterior hairline incision. The submental access incision is still placed approximately 1 cm behind the submental crease and is approximately 3 cm in length.

Extent of Undermining

Extended undermining in a subcutaneous plane is recommended for successful release of facial ligaments and zones of fusion.[10] In the cheek, undermining should be performed to just lateral to the zygomaticus major muscle to allow for access to the mobile SMAS. Limited, or minimal, undermining of the skin is unlikely to successfully treat the amount of laxity and redundancy and will place undue tension on the closure. The cheek flaps are extended down into the neck in a preplatysmal plane and then joined in the submental area. Care is taken during dissection over the sternocleidomastoid muscle (SCM) to avoid injury of the great auricular nerve in the region of the Osturk triangle.[11] To get full mobilization of the skin flaps, it is important to consider release of the mandibular septum and mandibular ligament, which allow easier access to the submental area. Release of these structures can decrease tethering around the jawline.

Hemostasis should be meticulously maintained throughout dissection. Bipolar cautery is preferred over monopolar because of less heat transmission to surrounding tissues and therefore less risk of facial nerve neuropraxia.

Lipodystrophy of the submental fat is common in MWL patients. Access to the neck with a submental incision provides excellent visualization of the platysma. Complete through-and-through undermining in the neck allows the surgeon to redrape the neck skin, and provides for direct excision and contouring of pre-platysmal and sub-platysmal fat.

Fat Transfer

In recent years, the popularity of fat grafting has revolutionized plastic surgery, in particular facial aesthetics and rejuvenation. The contributions by Rohrich and Pessa,[12] with their descriptions of the facial fat compartments laid the groundwork for plastic surgeons to isolate and selectively augment distinct areas of the face.

Fat injections in conjunction with facelift are vital in the MWL population. The cheeks are deflated, which creates an even more prominent fold of tissue over the nasolabial crease.[13] There is a loss of midface volume and often an accentuation of the buccal hollows. The temporal hollows often need to be addressed as well.

Filling of the deep malar, nasolabial, and oral commissure areas is beneficial. In a recent survey of American Society of Plastic Surgery members, 85% use fat grafting in combination with facelift. The most common areas were the deep malar, lower lid, cheek, and nasolabial fold.[14] On average, it takes more fat in the MWL patient to achieve full correction, even twice as much as would normally be injected in a non-MWL patient. This is especially true in the deep malar fat compartment, which helps to blend the lid/cheek transition.

Processing of the fat is a topic that continues to evolve. Traditional options include gravity separation, centrifugation, and separation on Telfa or cheesecloth. Some newer methods of fat processing include the Revolve System (Allergan, Dublin, Ireland), and Puregraft (Puregraft, Solana Beach, CA). A full comparison of different fat-processing methods goes beyond the scope of this article. There is not one method that has proven superior to others, so selection should be based on surgeon comfort, experience, cost, and familiarity of the operating room (OR) staff with different preparation techniques.

Treatment of the Superficial Musculoaponeurotic System

The topic of treating the SMAS is ongoing. There are 4 main approaches: SMAS plication, SMASectomy, extended SMAS flap with elevation, and composite flap. Although it is not clear in the literature that any one of these methods is superior for long-term correction, what is clear is that the SMAS needs to be addressed in some manner. Zins performs an extended SMAS, SMASectomy, and SMAS plication on MWL patients depending on anatomy. He suggests that wide skin undermining is more critical than the technique of SMAS repositioning in regard to the final result.[4] Rohrich treats the SMAS either obliquely or vertical depending on the patient's anatomy. He believes MWL patients usually require SMASectomy to remove redundant SMAS.[5]

It stands to reason that each patient's facial structure and soft tissues should be individually assessed. Regardless of method, elevation of the skin flaps needs to be performed medially enough to allow for exposure and manipulation of the mobile SMAS. Sufficient elevation of the SMAS is difficult to accomplish if adequate release is not performed. Patients with a long and narrow face with midface volume loss may benefit more from an SMAS plication or an extended SMAS flap, both of which recruit more SMAS into the midface. On the other hand, patients with shorter or fuller faces may benefit more from SMASectomy to remove some of the redundant SMAS and limit the amount of tissue being recruited to the midface.

Treatment of the Neck

Skin excess and neck laxity, whether skin alone or a combination of skin and muscle, is almost universal in MWL patients. When the soft tissues of the neck go through expansion followed by rapid deflation through weight loss, they are not elastic enough to contract to their previous position. This loss of elasticity causes them to pull away from the underlying neck structures, which results in sagging of the skin and an obtuse cervicomental angle. In a similar fashion, platysmal bands can become more visible and contribute to the appearance of accelerated aging. Platysmal banding is most common in thin necks.

Wide undermining with submental access is necessary with significant skin laxity or redundancy. Undermining the neck in a subcutaneous preplatysmal plane allows the skin to easily redrape and minimizes tension. Any excess preplatysmal fat can be easily visualized and directly excised and contoured.

The next decision that has to be made is whether or not to open the platysma. Although opening the submental region increases morbidity, the degree of improvement it offers for these patients likely outweighs the risks. Direct contouring of the subplatysmal fat can be performed at this time. Caution must be exercised during this maneuver to avoid overresection and creation of a submental hollowed out appearance. A good rule of thumb is to resect subplatysmal fat only to the level of the digastric muscles, and only if indicated.

Platysmal laxity is almost always present medially, requiring midline platysmaplasty. Feldman[15,16] elegantly described the corset platysmaplasty and believes platysmal laxity is best treated medially. The corset platysmaplasty involves a 2-layer running closure of the midline platysma with the second layer outside the first layer incorporating slightly more muscle than the first layer.[15,16] The suture begins in the submental area of the chin, extends down to the thyroid cartilage, and then back up to the chin. Other investigators advocate for a single layer of buried interrupted stitches to approximate the platysma muscle.[17] Suture choice is usually a long-lasting absorbable material, such as Polydioxanone, or a permanent stitch like Mersilene (Ethicon, Somerville, NJ).

Additional platysma laxity can be treated laterally by performing a lateral platysma window to better define the mandibular border. The platysma window involves creating a flap of platysma from a point 1 finger breadth below the angle of the mandible and 1 finger breadth anterior to the SCM and plication to the posterior mastoid fascia.[18]

Feldman and others also describe a suturing technique from the chin to the mastoid in an attempt to further define the lower mandibular border.[15,19] This is a variant of spanning sutures, but avoids abnormal tension in contours created by the latter.

POSTOPERATIVE MANAGEMENT

The postoperative management of the MWL facelift patient is essentially the same as for non-MWL patients.

The use of closed suction drains in the neck is recommended for at least 24 hours, and longer if indicated by output. There is little downside to leaving a drain in for an additional day to avoid a seroma that might take weeks or months to fully resolve.

Although ideally addressed preoperatively, these patients may be nutritionally challenged. They should resume a normal diet as soon as possible and consume adequate levels of protein to help ensure proper wound healing.

Early ambulation is encouraged; however, patients are instructed not to strain, bend over, or participate in highly aerobic activity for at least 2 weeks.

ADJUNCT PROCEDURES

Adjunct procedures to facelift are common and include, but are not limited to the following:

- Browlift.
- Blepharoplasty.
- Earlobe reduction.
- Lip lift.
- Direct excision of nasolabial folds. Although not appropriate for all MWL patients, direct excision of the nasolabial folds can be considered as a secondary procedure in those with residual deep nasolabial folds. Excision should be performed as a staged procedure. This can, and should, be discussed with the patient preoperatively. A well-placed incision

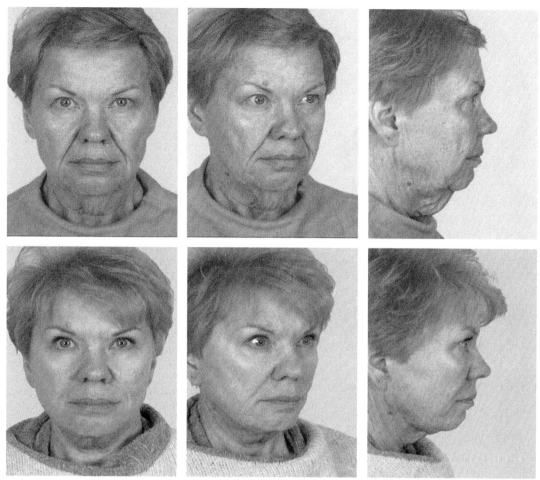

Fig. 1. A 55-year-old woman with a history of 100-pound weight loss by dieting (*above*). She underwent a 2-staged procedure: an extended SMAS facelift combined with an upper eyelid blepharoplasty and platysmaplasty, followed by a direct excision of nasolabial fold and CO_2 laser resurfacing 8 months later. Although the patient would benefit from revision on the cervical region, the patient was content with the results achieved and did not desire additional procedures. She is seen 16 months after the facelift (*below*). (*From* Couto RA, Waltzman JT, Tadisina KK, et al. An objective assessment of facial rejuvenation after massive weight loss. Aesthetic Plast Surg 2015;39(6):851; with permission.)

and meticulous closure can result in a very acceptable cosmetic outcome.

- Laser/chemical resurfacing. Resurfacing areas of the face that have not undermined is safe. If performing at the same time, care must be taken over the areas of skin flap elevation. Staged resurfacing allows for treatment of the entire face with less concern for compromising skin flaps.

Combining procedures can be convenient and beneficial for the patient; however, this needs to be weighed against the amount of time spent under anesthesia. Longer surgeries carry higher morbidity and risk to the patient, as well as surgeon fatigue. Risk for deep venous thrombosis, among others, needs to be assessed and treated appropriately. For some patients, a staged

approach can be the safest. In a recent article, Kappos and colleagues[20] showed that patient satisfaction was higher with combined procedures versus facelift alone.

STAGED AND REVISION PROCEDURES

The possibility of a staged or revision procedure should be discussed preoperatively with all MWL patients. Although not specifically written for MWL patients, Rawlani and Mustoe[8] described their approach to a planned staged facelift in patients with severe preoperative laxity. Most of the skin laxity is addressed in the first surgery, but there may be areas in which the degree of skin excess, or loss of skin elasticity, is too great to obtain full correction. Additionally, even in the best of

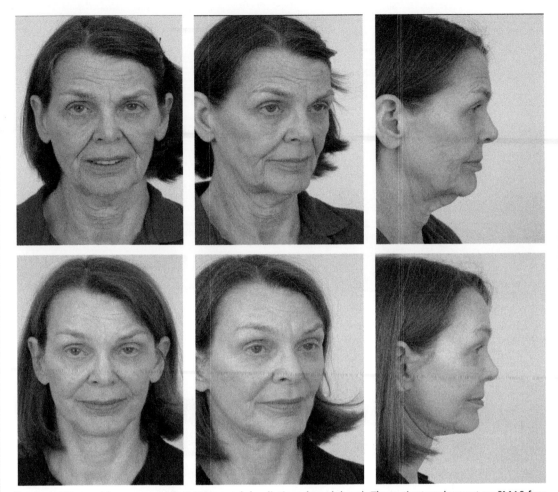

Fig. 2. A 64-year-old woman who lost 108 pounds by dieting alone (*above*). The patient underwent an SMAS face-lift combined with an endoscopic brow lift and platysmaplasty was performed. Five months later, she underwent direct nasolabial fold excision, perioral phenol-croton oil peel, and CO_2 laser resurfacing as revision procedure. She is seen 12 months after the rhytidectomy (*below*). (*From* Couto RA, Waltzman JT, Tadisina KK, et al. An objective assessment of facial rejuvenation after massive weight loss. Aesthetic Plast Surg 2015;39(6):852; with permission.)

conditions there is always some degree of expected recurrence. In these cases, a staged approach can be the most helpful. The cost of the second procedure also should be discussed with the patient before surgery so there is no confusion.

Revision procedures also should be discussed preoperatively. These procedures can include the following:

- Direct excision of nasolabial folds
- Laser/chemical resurfacing
- Scar revision
- Fat grafting

Figs. 1–4 show representative before-and-after pictures of MWL patients who underwent facelifting surgery. All patients experienced at least a 100-pound weight loss. Adjunct procedures, when performed, are mentioned.

MANAGEMENT OF COMPLICATIONS

The management of complications is no different in the MWL population from in the non-MWL population. Hematoma is perhaps the most common and serious early complication after facelift surgery. Hypertension is the most common cause of hematoma.[21] Protocols including clonidine patches, aggressive treatment of postoperative hypertension with labetalol and hydralazine, and keeping the blood pressure less than 140 mm Hg systolic have been documented to decrease this incidence.[22,23] Expeditious identification and treatment of hematomas usually has no long-term consequence to the patient's postoperative course or final outcome. Failure to identify or bring the patient back to the OR for a washout can result in further complications, such as discomfort, flap

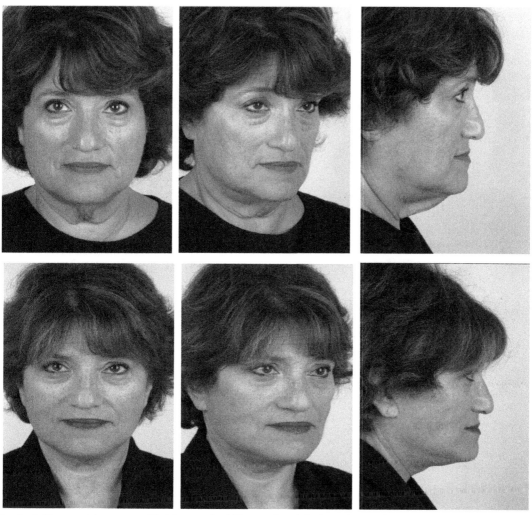

Fig. 3. A 57-year-old woman with history of a 100-pound weight loss after undergoing gastric bypass surgery (*above*). She underwent an extended SMAS facelift and transconjunctival lower lid blepharoplasty. She is seen on her 8-month follow-up photograph (*below*). (*From* Couto RA, Waltzman JT, Tadisina KK, et al. An objective assessment of facial rejuvenation after massive weight loss. Aesthetic Plast Surg 2015;39(6):853; with permission.)

necrosis, prolonged inflammatory response, asymmetry, induration, and patient dissatisfaction.

Seromas can be usually serially aspirated in the office, and if necessary a drain replaced.

Flap necrosis is probably the most feared complication after facelift. Abstinence from smoking for at least 4 weeks preoperatively greatly reduces the chances of flap necrosis, and facelift surgery should not be performed on patients who are actively smoking or using nicotine-containing products.[24] Urine cotinine can be used as an effective screening method in previous smokers. Treatment with local wound care is the mainstay of treatment. Hyperbaric oxygen therapy, if available, also may be useful in minimizing the amount of tissue loss. Early excision and advancing the skin

flaps should not be attempted, as this will only put more tension on an already compromised flap.

Nerve injury after facelift, although rare, can be devastating for the patient and distressing for the surgeon. The most commonly injured sensory nerve is the great auricular nerve, as it passes over the SCM. Injury results in numbness to the lower half of the ear. If complete transection of the nerve is witnessed, it should be repaired immediately under loupe magnification. Unwitnessed partial injury or edema around the nerve will often improve with time, and full sensation return in a matter of weeks to several months.

The most common symptomatic facial nerve injury is the marginal mandibular nerve, as it passes over the mandible and crosses superficial

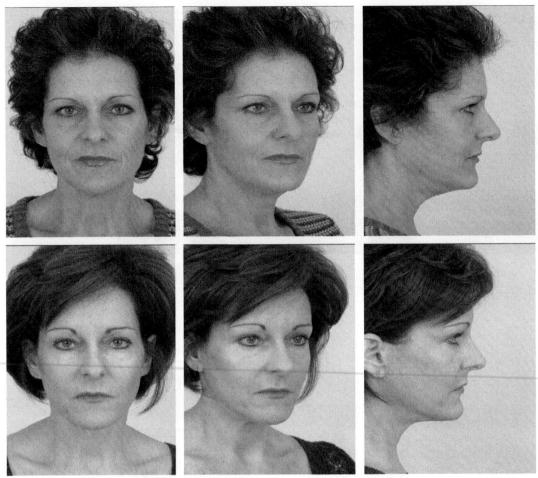

Fig. 4. A 48-year-old woman who lost 110 pounds after undergoing gastric bypass surgery (*above*). The patient underwent an extended SMAS facelift combined with endoscopic browlift, periocular laser resurfacing, and fat injections to the cheeks, nasolabial folds, infraorbital rims, and lips. A revision of endoscopic brow lift was performed 10 months later. She is shown 32 months after the rhytidectomy (*below*). (*From* Couto RA, Waltzman JT, Tadisina KK, et al. An objective assessment of facial rejuvenation after massive weight loss. Aesthetic Plast Surg 2015;39(6):854; with permission.)

to the facial vessels. Injury causes weakening of the lip depressors on that side and results in a deformity when opening the mouth, smiling, or grimacing. Staying superficial to the SMAS/platysma in this region, and avoidance of heavy use of monopolar electrocautery in the area limit the chances of complete transection. Partial nerve injuries often achieve full recovery, but can take weeks to months.

The most commonly injured facial nerve branch is actually considered to be the buccal branch; however, due to cross-innervation and significant arborization, these injuries are often short lived or completely asymptomatic. Zygomatic nerve injuries can occur just inferior to the zygomaticus major muscle during sub-SMAS dissection in the region of the McGregor patch.[25] Cervical nerve

injuries are most common, as the nerve exits from the inferior aspect of the parotid. The frontal branch nerve injuries are most common within 2 cm cephalad of the zygomatic arch, where it is just deep to the temporoparietal fascia.[26]

Widened scars are best prevented at the time of surgery by avoiding high amounts of tension on the skin flap during closure. Scar revision is often possible after complete healing has taken place. Planning is critical because there will be a defect once the scar is excised that will need to be closed under minimal tension to avoid recurrence. Fractionated CO_2 laser resurfacing can be a useful adjunct to help scars symptomatically and cosmetically.

Bunching of the skin can occur most commonly around the sideburn or behind the ear. Most of the time these areas will settle after several months as the tissues relax. Occasionally revision of excess skin may be required to allow for a smooth closure. This can usually be performed in the office under local anesthesia.

CONTROVERSIES

Most of the controversy in facelift surgery has to do with treatment of the SMAS and whether or not to open the neck. For treatment of the SMAS, it seems reasonable that a bilamellar approach is most appropriate. Treating the skin and SMAS separately and in their own vectors of pull helps to address the discrepant skin excess in MWL patients. The argument for a unilamellar approach, like a composite facelift, is that it enhances blood supply and combines the benefits of resistance to suture tearing and less stress relaxation.[8]

Opening the neck and manipulation of the underlying structures is a decision that is best made on a case-by-case basis. There are some who will advocate that opening the neck is never necessary, and others will say that it always needs to be opened. In the MWL population, the small increase in complications that results from opening the submental area is outweighed by the benefit that results.

SUMMARY

Similar to other areas of the body after MWL, the face and neck are not immune. Deflation of the tissues and loss of skin elasticity can result in the appearance of accelerated facial aging. Surgical facial rejuvenation can successfully be performed on the MWL patient with several modifications. These include the following:

- Proper preoperative counseling and expectation management regarding staged or ancillary procedures.
- Extended incisions along the posterior hairline.
- Wide undermining of the face and neck to allow for mobilization of excess skin and access to the mobile SMAS.
- Midface volumizing with selective placement of fat injections into the deep malar compartment.
- Treatment of the SMAS with plication, excision, or flap elevation.
- Treatment of the platysma in the midline, laterally, or both.
- Evaluation for adjunct procedures.

REFERENCES

1. Herman CK, Hoschander AS, Wong A. Post-bariatric body contouring. Aesthet Surg J 2015;35(6): 672–87.
2. Sclafani AP. Restoration of the jawline and the neck after bariatric surgery. Facial Plast Surg 2005;21(1): 28–32.
3. Stuzin JM. Restoring facial shape in face lifting: the role of skeletal support in facial analysis and midface soft-tissue repositioning (Baker Gordon symposium cosmetic series). Plast Reconstr Surg 2006; 191:362–77.
4. Couto RA, Waltzman JT, Tadisina KK, et al. An objective assessment of facial rejuvenation after massive weight loss. Aesthetic Plast Surg 2015;39(6):847–55.
5. Narasimhan K, Ramanadham S, Rohrich RJ. Face lifting in the massive weight loss patient: modifications of our technique for this population. Plast Reconstr Surg 2015;135(2):397–405.
6. Lupoli R, Lembo E, Saldalamacchia G, et al. Bariatric surgery and long-term nutritional issues. World J Diabetes 2017;8(11):464–74.
7. Capon T. Standardised anatomical alignment of the head in a clinical photography studio. A comparison between the Frankfort Horizontal and the natural head position. J Vis Commun Med 2016;39(3–4): 105–11.
8. Rawlani V, Mustoe TA. The staged face lift: addressing the biomechanical limitations of the primary rhytidectomy. Plast Reconstr Surg 2012;130(6): 1305–14
9. Pannucci CJ, MacDonald JK, Ariyan S, et al. Benefits and risks of prophylaxis for deep venous thrombosis and pulmonary embolus in plastic surgery: a systematic review and meta-analysis of controlled trials and consensus conference. Plast Reconstr Surg 2016;137(2):709–30.
10. Alghoul M, Bitik O, McBride J, et al. Relationship of the zygomatic facial nerve to the retaining ligaments of the face: the Sub-SMAS danger zone. Plast Reconstr Surg 2013;131(2):245e–52e.
11. Ozturk CN, Ozturk C, Huettner F, et al. A failsafe method to avoid injury to the great auricular nerve. Aesthet Surg J 2014;34(1):16–21.
12. Rohrich RJ, Pessa JE. The fat compartments of the face: anatomy and clinical implications for cosmetic surgery. Plast Reconstr Surg 2007;119(7):2219–27.
13. Yousif NJ, Gosain A, Sanger JR, et al. The nasolabial fold: a photogrammetric analysis. Plast Reconstr Surg 1994;93(1):70–7.
14. Sinno S, Mehta K, Simmons C, et al. Current trends in facial rejuvenation: an assessment of ASPS members utilization of fat grafting during facelifting. Plast Reconstr Surg 2015;136(5):141.
15. Feldman JJ. Corset platysmaplasty. Plast Reconstr Surg 1990;85(3):333–43.

16. Feldman JJ. Neck lift my way: an update. Plast Reconstr Surg 2014 Dec;134(6):1173–83.

17. Rohrich RJ, Narasimhan K. Long-term results in face lifting: observational results and evolution of technique. Plast Reconstr Surg 2016;138(1):97–108.

18. Cruz RS, O'Reilly EB, Rohrich RJ. The platysma window: an anatomically safe, efficient, and easily reproducible approach to neck contour in the face lift. Plast Reconstr Surg 2012;129(5):1169–72.

19. Giampapa V, Bitzos I, Ramirez O, et al. Suture suspension platysmaplasty for neck rejuvenation revisited: technical fine points for improving outcomes. Aesthetic Plast Surg 2005;29(5):341 50 [discussion: 351–2].

20. Kappos EA, Temp M, Toth BA, et al. Validating facial aesthetic surgery results with FACE-Q. Plast Reconstr Surg 2017;139:839.

21. Baker DC, Stefani WA, Chiu ES. Reducing the incidence of hematoma requiring surgical evacuation following male rhytidectomy: a 30-year review of 985 cases. Plast Reconstr Surg 2005;116(7):1973–85 [discussion: 1986–7].

22. Beer GM, Goldscheider E, Weber A, et al. Prevention of acute hematoma after face-lifts. Aesthetic Plast Surg 2010;34(4):502–7.

23. Ramanadham SR, Mapula S, Costa C, et al. Evolution of hypertension management in face lifting in 1089 patients: optimizing safety and outcomes. Plast Reconstr Surg 2015;135(4):1037–43.

24. Carter BD, Abnet CC, Feskanich D, et al. Smoking and mortality—beyond established causes. N Engl J Med 2015;372(7):631–40.

25. Furnas DW. The retaining ligaments of the cheek. Plast Reconstr Surg 1989;83(1):11–6.

26. Roostaeian J, Rohrich RJ, Stuzin JM. Anatomical considerations to prevent facial nerve injury. Plast Reconstr Surg 2015;135(5):1318–27.

Common Complications and Management After Massive Weight Loss Patient Safety in Plastic Surgery

Omar E. Beidas, MD, Jeffrey A. Gusenoff, MD*

KEYWORDS

- Body contouring • Plastic surgery • Massive weight loss • Complications • Prevention
- Management

KEY POINTS

- Although complications after body contouring for the massive weight loss patient are common, most are minor and manageable on an outpatient basis.
- The major risk factor for complications in this population is related to body mass indices.
- The most common complications after body contouring are seroma and wound dehiscence.
- Careful preoperative evaluation and intraoperative measures can decrease the rate of complications or prevent them altogether.

INTRODUCTION

There has been a rapid rise in popularity of plastic surgery after massive weight loss (MWL), as evidenced by a year-on-year increase in procedures performed as reported by the American Society of Plastic Surgeons.[1] The commonly accepted definition of MWL is a loss of more than 50% of excess body weight above ideal body weight. Most patients achieve MWL by means of bariatric surgery, some by diet and exercise, and a select few with weight loss drugs. Regardless of the method of weight loss, these patients are at an increased risk of complications compared with the general plastic surgery population.

Although reporting of complications is ubiquitously inconsistent across plastic surgery, the complication rate can be as high as 50% in a series publishing results of body contouring after MWL. Fortunately for patients and physicians, most complications encountered are minor and treated on an outpatient basis. Many times, all that is required of the physician is a closer, possibly prolonged period of follow-up and patient reassurance. The purpose of this article is to give readers tips to decrease the severity—if not altogether prevent—these complications.

As discussed in this series, a careful preoperative evaluation is the first step in avoiding complications. Although the topic is covered extensively in Capla J, and Shikowitz-Behr L: Patient Evaluation and Surgical Staging, in this issue, certain salient points deserve mention because they correlate directly with complications. Specific aspects worth revisiting as part of the preoperative work-up include weight history, weight loss method, body mass index (BMI), medical comorbidities, nutrition assessment, and nicotine use.

Because weight and BMI are directly related, it is useful to ascertain a patient's maximum and current weights. Those who have lost more than 100 lb have the highest risk of wound

The authors have nothing to disclose.
Department of Plastic Surgery, University of Pittsburgh, 3380 Boulevard of the Allies, Suite 180, Pittsburgh, PA 15213, USA
* Corresponding author.
E-mail address: gusenoffa@upmc.edu

complications.[2] Additionally, a higher BMI value at time of initial consult or surgery is associated with an increased rate of complications.[3,4] Despite these data, strict BMI cutoffs are not recommended because they eliminate patients prior to a formal evaluation, and some of these patients may benefit from a functional procedure.

The method by which a patient achieved weight loss is pertinent because this can affect the patient's nutritional status. Most patients who present for body contouring after MWL have undergone bariatric surgery, so the plastic surgeon operating must be familiar with the various bariatric surgery procedures. Some weight loss surgeries have a malabsorptive component, which may make it difficult to maintain appropriate nutritional intake and lead to various deficiencies.

Nutritional deficiencies are common in the post–bariatric surgery patient, with up to half of patients having at least 1 deficiency despite supplementation.[5–7] The most common deficiency in weight loss patients is iron, reported in up to 50% in some studies. Other commonly reported deficiencies include vitamin B, vitamin D, and calcium.[8]

COMMON COMPLICATIONS

A requisite part of the consent process involves a face-to-face discussion between physician and patient outlining the complications. Patients should have a clear understanding of what it means to have a dehiscence, what exactly a seroma or fat necrosis is, and how it is usually managed. Although body contouring procedures have a lengthy list of possible complications, most of these are easily managed. Even the smallest of complications seems like a major setback to the patient, so up-front discussion of possible outcomes is appreciated and better tolerated.

Although patients undergoing multiple procedures in one stage tend to have a higher risk of complications, the per-procedure complication rate remains stable when comparing specific complications.[9] Patients should be instructed to call the physician's office at the first sign of any problem, so potential serious complications may be mitigated through early assessment and intervention. In the following section, common complications, ways to prevent them, and their management are discussed.

Wound Dehiscence/Delayed Wound Healing

Wound dehiscence is the most common complication after plastic surgery in the MWL patient, reported as up to 15% in some studies,[9] twice as common in the extremities than in the trunk.[10]

Fortunately, most of these can be managed on an outpatient basis with basic local wound care. The procedure with the highest risk of dehiscence is the lower body lift with buttock auto-augmentation, with the lateral thigh and midline back the areas at most risk. The next most common area for dehiscence is the upper thigh, likely secondary to motion, pressure with sitting, and the nature of the tension in the area combined with the moist, bacteria-rich environment of the groin. Similarly, any incision with a T-point junction is at risk of dehiscence due to the tension at the junction of the 2 incision lines.

Prevention

Rates of wound dehiscence can be decreased by avoiding undue tension on incision lines. Wound closure should be performed in at least 2 layers, reapproximating the superficial fascial system—as described by Lockwood[11]—and the dermis. Undermining is ill advised, so if wound dehiscence occurs, the wound is significantly smaller and more easily managed. Postoperatively, pressure should be avoided on the operated region to minimize tension on the area. Patients should refrain from lifting, pushing, or pulling items heavier than 5 kg for 6 weeks after surgery to decrease the risk of wound dehiscence. For lower body lift procedures, they should avoid bending over sharply for 3 weeks after surgery. For thighplasty, permanent sutures in the groin can decrease potential breakdown.

Management

Management of any dehiscence must take several factors into consideration, including but not limited to size and depth, acuity, patient factors, and operating room (OR) availability. Acuity is important because patients who present days after a dehiscence harbor bacteria that prohibit closure even in the OR, because a secondary infection is extremely likely. Size is pertinent because small wounds are best managed with packing rather than closure, whereas larger wounds may be amenable to closure or require negative pressure wound therapy. A large dehiscence causing exposure or presenting with necrosis of a large area may require débridement or vacuum-assisted closure therapy. These wounds can take months to heal.

Patient factors play a vital role, including a patient's nutrition as well as tolerance to local anesthetic and in-office procedures. A large, deep dehiscence should be considered a sign of malnutrition until proved otherwise. The patient should be screened for any nutrition deficiencies and levels of prealbumin and albumin checked. A dietician may be helpful in recommending appropriate sources of protein to hasten the wound healing process.

Finally, the acuity of the dehiscence is important because large wounds that have been open for less than 24 hours are amenable to reclosure with proper technique. The urgent nature of treating such a wound is the reason it is imperative that patients are told to call the physician's office immediately should they experience a major dehiscence. If a patient can tolerate local anesthesia, the wound may be irrigated with the antibiotic of choice and closed in layers over a drain in clinic. If patient or wound factors dictate the need for an OR, and one is readily available, the closure can be performed in the sterile setting of the OR. The availability of an OR, however, should not cause a substantial delay if a wound requires closure acutely. In such instances, the emergency department can be considered a secondary OR where proper instruments, lighting, medications, and staff are available to the surgical team. In any of these instances, the patient should be placed on a course of antibiotics of approximately 1-week duration. If a patient presents in a delayed fashion, or the wound is not amenable to closure due to a necrotic portion of tissue, the necrotic portion should be débrided and local wound care initiated. In large, extensive wounds, this may require use of negative pressure wound therapy until transitioned to traditional gauze dressing. Again, these patients should be screened for malnutrition and would be best served by seeing a dietitian.

Seroma

Seromas occur when a dead space is created and not closed down or drained adequately. It is a common complication with these procedures, with a prevalence of 5% to 15% in this population.[12,13] The most common site is the abdomen; other areas prone to accumulate fluid include the distal part of a brachioplasty, the distal part of a thighplasty, and the posterior midline in a lower body lift. Dead space is much smaller and, therefore, drains are often not needed when performing chest procedures.

Prevention
Many factors can play a role in development of seroma formation. Seroma can be circumvented with careful surgical dissection, or use of drains, fibrin glue,[14,15] or progressive tension suture as described by Pollock and Pollock.[16] In the abdomen, the plane of dissection should be immediately on the abdominal wall fascia only in the location where rectus muscle plication is to be performed. Outside this region, some fatty tissue deep to Scarpa fascia should be left on the anterior abdominal wall to preserve lymphatics. Maintaining this tissue low on the abdominal wall remains controversial.[17]

Postoperative compression garments may aid in closing potential spaces for fluid collection. If drains are used, patients are seen weekly until all are removed. A common criterion for drain removal is output less than 30 mL over a 24-hour period, although some surgeons prefer to extend this criterion to 2 days. Drains are typically in place for 7 days to 14 days. Once drains are removed, patients may transition to a nonmedical compression garment of choice or can continue to use their postoperative compression dressing.

Management
A seroma is most easily recognized by a visible or palpable fluid wave subcutaneously. If readily available, an ultrasound can be used to detect as well as guide drainage of the collection. Unless this is available in the clinic, however, it is more cost effective to attempt manual drainage of a suspected area than to send a patient to a radiologist for drainage. If a seroma develops, it can be controlled with serial aspiration. A patient who requires an aspiration should be assessed weekly for reaspiration if needed. If after 3 rounds of aspiration, the fluid collection continues to reaccumulate, a seroma catheter can be placed.

If a drain is present yet output remains high after a few weeks, chemical sclerosis can be performed using doxycycline or bleomycin mixed with local anesthetic in the clinic. The drain is clamped and the patient is turned every 15 minutes for 1 hour to spread the antibiotic over all walls of the cavity. If this fails to close down the dead space, then the seroma can either be marsupialized or excised and closed over a drain.

Hematoma

Hematoma, although uncommon, can range from a small collection that may be left alone to an expanding one requiring operative intervention. Reported hematoma rates in the literature range from 1% to 20%[10,12,13,18] and is more frequent in men compared with women and in the trunk compared with the extremities. Risk factors for hematoma formation include sustained hypothermia below 35.6°C or an average temperature of 35.2°C.[18]

Prevention
The initial screen to reduce the risk of hematoma is to verify that a patient's blood pressure is under control during the preoperative visit. Undocumented or uncontrolled hypertension should be

managed in the preoperative period so that it does not cause a problem postoperatively. Postoperative hypertension, defined by an increased mean arterial pressure, has been shown to be a risk factor for hematoma.[19]

Intraoperatively, surgical technique is paramount to avoiding a hematoma. Incision lines and dissection planes can be infiltrated with epinephrine solution to decrease vascularity of the region. Various methods are available to obtain hemostasis, whether with use of electrocautery, hemoclips, or sutures. Large vessels should almost certainly be clipped or suture ligated, especially those emanating from the abdominal wall fascia, because these are likely to cause a problem postoperatively. Irrigation should be done with warm fluid to avoid vessel spasm and manual friction should be used directly on the exposed tissues; these maneuvers may uncover an early clot that could otherwise dislodge and lead to a bleed postoperatively. A low mean arterial pressure in the last 2 hours of a procedure is associated with increased hematoma rates. Therefore, at the time of hemostasis, the surgery and anesthesia teams should coordinate to avoid hypotension. A squeeze test along incision lines can reveal vessels that may have spasmed.[20] For abdominal wall procedures, a Valsalva maneuver may be used to simulate increased pressure.

Management

A small hematoma can be monitored closely to ensure it does not enlarge or become infected. Large hematomas are generally best evacuated because, if left alone, they can cause contour deformities in the long term, require prolonged drains, and are aggravating to patients. After 7 days to 10 days, clotted blood liquefies and is absorbed by the body or, alternatively, can be aspirated in clinic.

Any expanding hematoma should be promptly evacuated and controlled in the operating room. Although a hematoma is not prevented by drain placement, a rapid increase in red bloody output can be a harbinger of a hematoma. A patient may show signs or symptoms of blood loss, such as decreased blood pressure, decreased urine output, or increased heart rate. On physical examination, an asymmetric contour may be noted between sides or ecchymosis and/or pain over an indurated area. It is important that dressings are taken down and the suspected region assessed, especially in the extremities where neurovascular compromise is possible due to the increased pressure in the cylindrical compartment.

A rapidly expanding hematoma causing systemic signs, as described previously, is a surgical emergency and the patient should be taken to the OR without delay. Resuscitative measures should be initiated until blood pressure stabilizes, beginning with a 2-L bolus of fluid followed by packed red blood cells as needed. Most times, this is a technical error and a bleeding vessel is discovered on exploration of the wound. Although there may be an obvious arterial or venous source of bleeding, there may be a diffuse ooze from all wound edges secondary to the administration of chemoprophylaxis for venous thromboembolism. Vessels should be clipped or suture ligated and the wound copiously irrigated to find any other possible sources of bleeding. Hemostatic agents, such as a fibrin sealant or thrombin spray, may be used in the wound bed.

Surgical Site Infection

Surgical site infection (SSI) can range from a mild cellulitis that responds to a course of oral antibiotics to a raging infection requiring operative débridement, intravenous antibiotics, and protracted healing. Reported rates of SSI in the literature range from 5% to 8%.

Prevention

Many preventative measures are in place to decrease the risk of infection. The Surgical Care Improvement Project (SCIP) has become the cornerstone of infection management. An antibiotic appropriate for the patient and procedure should be administered within the recommended time frame and redosed according to its half-life. Studies have shown no benefit to continuing antibiotics past 24 hours after the end of a procedure.[21,22] Despite this high-level evidence,[23] many surgeons use antibiotics past 24 hours or until drains are removed. Shaving should be avoided in the 48 hours leading up to a procedure and, if not done by the patient before this time frame, clippers should be used on the day of surgery before skin preparation.[24] The skin site should be cleansed using chlorhexidine-alcohol, because it is more effective than povidone-iodine.[25] Literature to support recommendations for large body contouring cases is, however, lacking.

Management

SSI generally occurs after the first postoperative week or can be delayed if antibiotic use is prolonged. Early signs of an infection, such as cellulitis, can be treated with oral antibiotics. Given the high prevalence of methicillin-resistant *Staphylococcus aureus*, first-line choice in a patient without a sulfonamide allergy should be trimethoprim/sulfamethoxazole (Bactrim). In a patient with an allergy or who failed Bactrim treatment, clindamycin should be considered. Some wounds may require incision and drainage along with antibiotic therapy; fortunately, many of these can be performed under local anesthesia in the clinic.

If an implant is in or near the locale of an SSI, treatment must be initiated expeditiously to prevent seeding of the foreign body. If the infection has reached the implant, then removal with irrigation is indicated. Replacement of an implant is not recommended but left to the discretion of the surgeon.[26]

Nonsurgical Site or Systemic Infection

A variety of sites outside the surgical field are at risk of infection. Patients can develop a postoperative urinary tract, thoracic, intestinal, or systemic infection (sepsis), among others.

Prevention
If a Foley catheter was used, it should be removed within 48 hours, barring any indication to leave it in place. Pneumonia is uncommon postoperatively in body contouring patients; however, patients should be screened for risk factors preoperatively and optimized accordingly. Those with preoperative risk factors or those undergoing abdominal surgery—making them more likely to splint breathing postoperatively—should be encouraged to go home with an incentive spirometer.

Management
A urinary tract infection is generally associated with prolonged catheter usage. Recommended treatment is culture and Gram stain of the urine along with removal or replacement of the catheter. Broad-spectrum antibiotics are initiated, after which antibiotics should be tailored based on culture results. This is extremely rare in the body-contouring population because these are mobile patients who do not require bladder drainage for prolonged periods of time.

Pneumonia is treated based on symptoms, with outpatient antibiotic management for mild cases or admission to a hospital with intravenous antibiotics for patients exhibiting systemic symptoms.

Due to the pervasive use of antibiotic therapy after plastic surgery procedures, despite studies proving no benefit, there has been an increased rate of intestinal *Clostridium difficile* infection. SCIP guidelines recommend that antibiotics should not be continued for longer than 24 hours, and studies have shown an almost 7-fold increase in *C difficile* rates in patients who receive antibiotic prophylaxis discordant with these guidelines.[27]

If any localized infection has progressed so far as to cause systemic symptoms, the patient should be admitted to a hospital, pan-cultured, and started on intravenous antibiotics. In patients without allergies, broad-spectrum coverage is initiated using vancomycin and piperacillin/tazobactam (Zosyn).

Lymphedema

After any operative procedure, patients may exhibit signs of lower extremity edema due to a multitude of factors, most commonly due to a combination of fluid overload and postoperative immobility. This may become more evident 2 weeks to 3 weeks later as the patient becomes increasingly active but lymphatic drainage has not caught up. Dependent edema should not persist past the 8-week mark. Although it has been shown that thighplasty after MWL alters the lymphatic drainage of the lower extremity,[28] the true rate of permanent edema—or lymphedema—after body contouring is unknown. In the thigh, risk factors for lymphedema are a vertical incision, male gender, and hypothyroidism.[29]

Prevention
Lower extremity edema can be common in the MWL patient, and careful preoperative evaluation must rule out preexisting vascular disease, especially in the patient considering thighplasty.[30] It is also important to recognize the difference between lymphedema and lipedema, which often are confused.[31] Lipedema presents as symmetric adiposity of the lower extremity from groin to ankle. The sine qua non of lipedema is an abrupt line of demarcation at the level of the ankle, and the adiposity does not affect the foot. In addition, there is associated pain of the subcutaneous tissues. A list of differences is presented in **Table 1**.

Intraoperatively, care must be taken to avoid disrupting lymphatic drainage of nearby sites. This means avoidance of deep resection in the axilla during a brachioplasty and similarly the inguinal region during a thighplasty or abdominoplasty.

Management
Any evidence of lower extremity edema should be investigated. History should focus on calf pain or cramping, shortness of breath, or chest pain. Physical examination should check for laterality, pain, pitting, and Homan sign.

Unilateral or asymmetric swelling is a cause of concern for deep vein thrombosis (DVT); bilateral or symmetric swelling is generally dependent swelling or lymphedema. If a DVT is not high on the differential or ruled out by ultrasound, then conservative measures for dependent edema are instituted. Initial therapy consists of elevation of extremities and compression or wraps from foot to groin. This protocol should be continued up to

Table 1
Differences between lymphedema and lipedema

	Lymphedema	Lipedema
Etiology of edema	Lymphatic disorder	Pathologic fatty deposits
Laterality	Unilateral or bilateral	Bilateral
Foot edema	Yes	No
Stemmer sign	Positive	Negative
Pitting edema	Yes	No
Pain	No	Yes

8 weeks. If the edema persists at this point, the patient should be referred to a lymphedema specialist for management. Edema that perseveres for 1 year is unlikely to reverse and be permanent.

Suture Extrusion

Although common in body contouring procedures, suture extrusion is usually a minor complication that is prevented with attention to detail and treated with local wound care.

Prevention

Meticulous operative technique is the best prevention for suture extrusion. When using suture near the dermis, one must be sure to bury knots. Suture ends should be cut with short tails to avoid spitting or irritation at the knot. Barbed suture offers time efficiency[32] but must be handled differently from standard suture. Barbed sutures must not come into contact with sponges or towels because they pick up strands that can create a foreign body reaction when sewn in.[33] Additionally, if used to close skin, this type of suture should be placed in the deeper dermis. Permanent braided suture should not be used in thin areas, such as the axilla and groin, because it can extrude more easily.

Management

Suture extrusion is generally easy to identify and manage. An impending extrusion can be identified by erythema, ecchymosis, blistering, drainage, or a combination of these along the incision line. A braided or monofilament suture that is extruding usually slowly exits through the skin without causing a wound dehiscence. Sometimes, this requires trimming the suture tail in question flush with the skin until the knot surfaces. Barbed suture, however, acts differently and often causes wound breakdown in the problem area. The exposed portion of the suture must be located with forceps and cut, or else the wound does not heal.

Fat Necrosis

Fat necrosis is a result of decreased vascularity to fatty tissue. Fortunately, it is a benign and usually self-limiting complication in body contouring. The most common sites for fat necrosis are the breast and abdomen.

Prevention

The key to avoiding fat necrosis is to ensure that all fatty tissue remains well perfused. Care must be taken to not place sutures in a manner that strangulates adipose tissue. When resecting tissue, large protruding mounds of fat should not be left hanging, because the blood supply to this region may be tenuous. Similarly, if performing autoaugmentation of the breast or buttocks using dermoglandular or adipose flaps, these must be raised with adequate thickness, width, and length.

Management

Fat necrosis is identified as hard, palpable lumps subcutaneously, commonly along the scar line. Treatment consists of observation because these areas usually resolve spontaneously with time. Areas in the breast may be concerning and can be sent for ultrasonography to rule out a mass. If the lump persists at 1 year and bothers the patient, the area can be excised in clinic.

Venous Thromboembolism

DVT/pulmonary embolism is uncommon but potentially catastrophic. Many thromboembolic events are preventable with appropriate prophylaxis, yet a survey of approximately 600 plastic surgeons performing body contouring procedures showed that more than one-third of surgeons use no chemical prophylaxis.[34] Although no guidelines currently exist for the plastic surgery patient, surgeons should refer to the 2005 Caprini score.[35]

Postoperative Dissatisfaction

Patients may be dissatisfied for many reasons; however, the most common ones encountered in MWL patients are standing tissue cones at incision ends, recurrent skin laxity, and asymmetry.

Prevention

As in many surgical evaluations, it is essential to discuss all possible outcomes with patients preoperatively. A thorough discussion of the risks prepare patients should they experience such a result. This conversation should be incorporated into the consent and serves to manage patient expectations. It is helpful to review the surgeon's revision policy at this time so that patients are aware of their responsibilities.

Management

A dissatisfied patient requires additional time during visits and repetitive reassurance. Asymmetries and standing tissue cones should be monitored for at least 6 months before proceeding with a revision, because many of these initial issues resolve with time. Many of these problems require minor revisions, although sometimes recurrent skin laxity may need a full revision of the previous operation. Patients who have yet to undergo further stages can opt to have these revisions performed in the same operative setting to avoid clinic revisions.

SUMMARY

Body contouring procedures are fraught with complications; many of these are manageable in the office setting. In all cases, it is best to manage a patient's expectations up-front rather than after a complication occurs. Knowledge of how to prevent and manage complications in this patient population is paramount, and the unexperienced surgeon should not tackle these cases without considerable experience.

REFERENCES

1. Plastic Surgery Statistics. American Society of Plastic Surgeons. Available at: https://www.plasticsurgery.org/news/plastic-surgery-statistics. Accessed January 17, 2018.
2. Constantine RS, Davis KE, Kenkel JM. The effect of massive weight loss status, amount of weight loss, and method of weight loss on body contouring outcomes. Aesthet Surg J 2014;34(4):578–83.
3. Chetta MD, Aliu O, Tran BA, et al. Complications in body contouring stratified according to weight loss method. Plast Surg (Oakv) 2016;24(2):103–6.
4. Coon D, Gusenoff JA, Kannan N, et al. Body mass and surgical complications in the postbariatric reconstructive patient: analysis of 511 cases. Ann Surg 2009;240(3):397–401.
5. Halverson JD. Metabolic risk of obesity surgery and long-term follow-up. Am J Clin Nutr 1992;55(2 Suppl):602S–5S.
6. van der Beek ES, Monpellier VM, Eland I, et al. Nutritional deficiencies in gastric bypass patients; incidence, time of occurrence and implications for post-operative surveillance. Obes Surg 2015;25(5): 818–23.
7. Stein J, Stier C, Raab H, et al. Review article: the nutritional and pharmacological consequences of obesity surgery. Aliment Pharmacol Ther 2014; 40(6):582–609.
8. Naghshineh N, O'Brien Coon D, McTigue K, et al. Nutritional assessment of bariatric surgery patients presenting for plastic surgery: a prospective analysis. Plast Reconstr Surg 2010;126(2):602–10.
9. Coon D, Michaels J 5th, Gusenoff JA, et al. Multiple procedures and staging in the massive weight loss population. Plast Reconstr Surg 2010;125(2):691–8.
10. Guest RA, Amar D, Czerniak S, et al. Heterogeneity in body contouring outcomes based research: the Pittsburgh body contouring complication reporting system. Aesthet Surg J 2017;38(1):60–70.
11. Lockwood TE. Superficial fascial system (SFS) of the trunk and extremities: a new concept. Plast Reconstr Surg 1991;87:1009–18.
12. Gusenoff JA, Coon D, Rubin JP. Implications of weight loss method in body contouring outcomes. Plast Reconstr Surg 2009;123(1):373–6.
13. Michaels J 5th, Coon D, Rubin JP. Complications in postbariatric body contouring: postoperative management and treatment. Plast Reconstr Surg 2011; 127(4):1693–700.
14. Grossman JA, Capraro PA. Long-term experience with the use of fibrin sealant in aesthetic surgery. Aesthet Surg J 2007;27:558–62.
15. Toman N, Buschmann A, Muehlberger T. Fibrin glue and seroma formation following abdominoplasty. Chirurg 2007;78:531–5.
16. Pollock TA, Pollock H. Progressive tension sutures: a technique to reduce local complications in abdominoplasty. Plast Reconstr Surg 2000;105:2583–6.
17. Friedman T, Coon D, Kanbour-Shakir A, et al. Defining the lymphatic system of the anterior abdominal wall: an anatomical study. Plast Reconstr Surg 2015;135(4):1027–32.
18. Cohen B, Meilik B, Weiss-Meilik A, et al. Intraoperative factors associated with postoperative complications in body contouring surgery. J Surg Res 2018; 221:24–9.
19. Farkas JP, Kenkel JM, Hatef DA, et al. The effect of blood pressure on hematoma formation with perioperative Lovenox in excisional body contouring surgery. Aesthet Surg J 2007;27(6):589–93.
20. Gusenoff JA. Prevention and management of complications in body contouring surgery. Clin Plast Surg 2014;41(4):805–18.
21. Phillips BT, Fourman MS, Bishawi M, et al. Are prophylactic postoperative antibiotics necessary for immediate breast reconstruction? results of a prospective randomized clinical trial. J Am Coll Surg 2016;222(6):1116–24.
22. Lewis A, Sen R, Hill TC, et al. Antibiotic prophylaxis for subdural and subgaleal drains. J Neurosurg 2017;126(3):908–12.
23. Hsu P, Bullocks J, Matthews M. Infection prophylaxis update. Semin Plast Surg 2006;20(4):241–8.

24. Tanner J, Woodings D, Moncaster K. Preoperative hair removal to reduce surgical site infection. Cochrane Database Syst Rev 2006;(3):CD004122.

25. Darouiche RO, Wall MJ Jr, Itani KM, et al. Chlorhexidine-alcohol versus povidone-iodine for surgical-site antisepsis. N Engl J Med 2010;361(1):18–26.

26. Spear SL, Howard MA, Boehmler JH, et al. The infected or exposed breast implant: management and treatment strategies. Plast Reconstr Surg 2004;113(6):1634–44.

27. Balch A, Wendelboe AM, Vesely SK, et al. Antibiotic prophylaxis for surgical site infections as a risk factor for infection with Clostridium difficile. PLoS One 2017;12(6):0179117.

28. Moreno CH, Neto HJ, Junior AH, et al. Thighplasty after bariatric surgery: evaluation of lymphatic drainage in lower extremities. Obes Surg 2008; 18(9):1160–4.

29. Shermak MA, Mallalieu J, Chang D. Does thighplasty for upper thigh laxity after massive weight loss require a vertical incision? Aesthet Surg J 2009;29(6):513–22.

30. Katzel EB, Nayar HS, Davenport MP, et al. The influence of preexisting lower extremity edema and venous stasis disease on body contouring outcomes. Ann Plast Surg 2014;73(4):365–70.

31. Okhovat JP, Alavi A. Lipedema: a review of the literature. Int J Low Extrem Wounds 2015;14(3):262–7.

32. Duscher D, Pollhammer MS, Wenny R, et al. Barbed sutures in body-contouring: outcome analysis of 695 procedures in 623 patients and technical advances. Aesthetic Plast Surg 2016;40(6):815–21.

33. Haenen FW, Van Cleemput M, Colpaert SD. A potential complication of barbed sutures preventing foreign body granulomas induced by surgical cloth particles. Aesthetic Plast Surg 2016;40(6): 972–3.

34. Clavijo-Alvarez JA, Pannucci CJ, Oppenheimer AJ, et al. Prevention of venous thromboembolism in body contouring surgery: a national survey of 596 ASPS surgeons. Ann Plast Surg 2011;66(3):228–32.

35. Caprini JA. Thrombosis risk assessment as a guide to quality patient care. Dis Mon 2005;51(2–3):70–8.

Moving?

Make sure your subscription moves with you!

To notify us of your new address, find your **Clinics Account Number** (located on your mailing label above your name), and contact customer service at:

Email: journalscustomerservice-usa@elsevier.com

800-654-2452 (subscribers In the U.S. & Canada)
314-447-8871 (subscribers outside of the U.S. & Canada)

Fax number: 314-447-8029

Elsevier Health Sciences Division
Subscription Customer Service
3251 Rivcrport Lane
Maryland Heights, MO 63043

*To ensure uninterrupted delivery of your subscription, please notify us at least 4 weeks in advance of move.

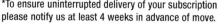

Printed and bound by CPI Group (UK) Ltd, Croydon, CR0 4YY

08/05/2025

01864740-0001